The Practical Guide to Herbal Medicines

The Practical Guide to Herbal Medicines

Formulas for Health and Wellness

DANIEL GAGNON
MS, RH (AHG)
Medical Herbalist

Botanical Research and Education Institute, Inc.
12 Palentine Road, Santa Fe, NM 87506

AUTHOR: Daniel Gagnon
EDITOR: Christa Weidner
EDITORIAL ASSISTANT: MaryEllen Collins
EDITORIAL CONSULTANT: Carole Tashel
GRAPHIC DESIGN: Janice St. Marie
COVER DESIGN AND LAYOUT: Matthew Roybal
BOOK & COVER ILLUSTRATIONS: Angela Werneke
  (©1995 Angela Werneke)

Cover shows California Poppy, Valerian, Passionflower, Oat and Orange peel as found in the Deep Sleep® formula.

©2016 Daniel J. Gagnon
ISBN: 978-0-9654530-2-8

ALL RIGHTS RESERVED. No part of this book may be reproduced in any form or by any electronic or mechanical means, including information storage and retrieval systems, without permission in writing from the author except by a reviewer who may quote brief passages in a review.

PUBLISHER
Botanical Research & Education Institute, Inc.
12 Palentine Road
Santa Fe, NM 87506

♻ Post-consumer recycled paper

Please note!

This book is designed to provide you with herbal healthcare options within the realm of herbal medicine. Keep in mind that the herbs listed in this book are mostly for preventive purposes and for health issues that do not require major medical intervention. This book is not intended to replace the expertise of a primary care practitioner or of a specialist. If the complaint you are treating is not getting better, or if it is getting worse, consult a doctor. The publisher, the author, and the editors do not assume any responsibility for any injury and/or damage to persons or property arising out of or related to any use of the material contained in this book. Additionally, the reader is advised to check the product information provided by the manufacturer to verify dosages, the method and duration of administration, as well as contraindications, side effects or warnings that may be associated with the therapeutic substances.

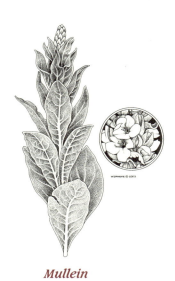

Mullein

About Daniel Gagnon

Daniel has been a practicing herbalist since 1976. Born in French Canada, his passion for helping others was born out of his own childhood health problems. His experience with conventional medical treatment of eczema, asthma and allergies motivated him to seek gentler, more effective healing modalities, which ultimately put him on the path to becoming an herbalist.

In 1979, he relocated to Santa Fe, New Mexico. There he furthered his studies in medical herbalism, pharmacognosy and related subjects at the Santa Fe College of Natural Medicine, the College of Santa Fe and the College of Pharmacy at the University of New Mexico. In 2004, he obtained his Bachelor of Science in Herbal Medicine from the North American College of Botanical Medicine in Albuquerque. In 2011 he completed his Masters Degree at the Scottish School of Herbal Medicine through the University of Wales. His thesis was on the antimicrobial effects of hops (*Humulus lupulus*) on methicillin-resistant *Staphylococcus aureus* (MRSA).

His goal is to educate the public and the medical profession about the practical, healing applications of herbal medicine. Health care professionals such as medical doctors, naturopaths, chiropractors and acupuncturists frequently call upon Daniel as an herbal consultant. He is the co-author of *Breathe Free*, a nutritional and herbal care book for the respiratory system. This book is the updated version of the national best-selling book *Liquid Herbal Drops in EveryDay Use* which sold more than 120,000 copies. Daniel regularly teaches seminars and classes on herbal therapeutics, both nationally and internationally.

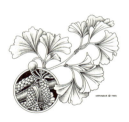

Ginkgo

Author's Introduction
About This Book

August 2015

Dear Herbal Medicine Enthusiast,

My goal in writing *The Practical Guide to Herbal Medicines*—whether you are just beginning to learn about herbs or you are already well on your way—is to provide you with the most practical, easy-reference guide to herbal medicines in the marketplace today. This book is an updated version of the national best-selling book, *Liquid Herbal Drops in Everyday Use,* which sold more than 120,000 copies. There are many books that generally explain "which herbs are good for what." This book helps you focus, in practical and specific terms, on which herbal formulas to take, what they are for, how they work, and how best to take them. It also warns you about contraindications, possible side effects and/or warnings.

The formulas listed in this book are ones that I have created over the past 30 years. I recommend them in my practice as a Medical Herbalist and in my role as a consultant to professional healthcare practitioners.

All the formulas in this book have an excellent track record in safety and efficacy. Over the years, some of them have been improved as a result of ongoing research and/or client feedback. These formulas are available at natural food markets, herb stores and natural pharmacies throughout the United States and Canada.

I welcome any of your suggestions or comments on how this book can be improved for the next edition. I also want to hear about your ideas on what additional herbs, health issues and formulas should be included in the next revision.

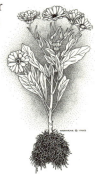

Calendula

8 Author's Introduction

I wish to thank all the people who have helped me create this book—professionals, retailers, consumers and colleagues. Their contributions have been invaluable. Many blessings for your suggestions and your insights.

I hope you find this resource guide useful. May it help and enlighten you in your quest for health.

Herbally Yours,

Daniel Gagnon

Daniel Gagnon

February 2016

I am amazed how quickly the first edition of *The Practical Guide to Herbal Medicines* has sold out. The good point about it is that it provided me with an opportunity to bring the book up to date. Small corrections, revisions, and deletions were made. Nothing major, just incremental improvements.

As always, I welcome your suggestions and comments. It is my hope that this book continues to provide you with practical herbal medicine suggestions in your quest for health.

In Health,

Daniel Gagnon

Daniel Gagnon

Contents

About Daniel Gagnon 6
Author's Introduction 7

CHAPTER 1: *The Ten Elements of Great Health* 12

CHAPTER 2: *Understanding Herbal Medicine*.. 17
What is herbal medicine and who uses it?.... 17
How does herbal medicine compare with current
    medical practices? 17
What healthcare benefits do herbs offer? 18
How do herbs differ from drugs? 19

CHAPTER 3: *Choosing The Herbal Products
    That Are Best for You*................. 21
Forms in which herbal products are available .. 21
Extracts offer the most therapeutic results ... 21
What are liquid herbal extracts?........... 21
Why herbalists recommend liquid
    herbal extracts 21
Liquid extract form preferable to capsules
    or tablets 23
How each type is made 24
Fresh herbs vs. dried herbs 25
Start with an alcohol and water extract 26
Understanding alcohol ratios in labeling 27
Alcohol content of an herbal extract dosage .. 27
Evaporating alcohol on a dose-by-dose basis . 28
How to avoid gluten in herbal products 28
Options on how to avoid alcohol in
    liquid herbal extracts 30
What is standardization?.. 30
Standardization and healing potential of herbs 32
Shelf life of different forms of herbs 34
Care and storage of liquid herbal extracts..... 34
When extracts "go bad" 35
Choosing organic herbs.................. 35

Criteria for choosing liquid extracts 35

Chapter 4: *Taking Herbal Medicine Extracts* 37

Choosing between formulas or single extracts .. 37
Using herbs for acute and chronic conditions .. 38
Best time of day to take herbs 39
When to stop taking herbs 39
Taking herbs for several different
   health problems 40
Taking herbs along with conventional drugs .. 41
Bitter taste and its healing benefits 41
Disguising the taste 42
Giving herbs to children 42
Getting children to take herbs 44
Giving herbs to pets 44
Comparing capsules to extracts and softgels .. 44
Equivalency of extracts and softgels
   to capsules 45

Chapter 5: *Deciding When to Avoid Certain Herbs* 46

Precautions during pregnancy or
   nursing 46
Single herbs and formulas to avoid
   during pregnancy 46
Single herbs and formulas to avoid while
   nursing 47
Herbs and prescription drugs 47
What are contraindications? 48
Herbs and side effects 48
What are warnings? 49
Contraindications of herbs 49
Possible side effects of herbs 49
Warnings for herbs 50

Discussing herbs with your doctor 51

CHAPTER 6: *Targeting Herbs for Specific Complaints* 52

What is herbal targeting? 52
Why target herbs for specific health
　　challenges? 52
How to get the most out of this chapter 53
Herbs for skin problems 53
Herbs for colds and flu 54
Herbs for smoking cessation 56
Herbs for allergies 57
Herbs for digestive problems 58
Herbs for women's reproductive system 59
Herbs for respiratory problems 60

CHAPTER 7: *Herbal Directory* 61

Alphabetical listing of herbal extracts from "A" (Acnetonic™) to "Y" (Yeast *ReLeaf*®) as well as information on single herbs found in formulas
[Cross-referenced by the Health Condition Index]

CHAPTER 8: *Single Herbs Used in Formulas* .. 86

CHAPTER 9: *Health Condition Index* 108

Alphabetical listing of health problems from "A" (Abdominal Pain) to "Y" (Yeast Infections)
[Cross-referenced to the Herbal Directory]

CHAPTER 10: *Common Name – Latin Name Index* 120

CHAPTER 11: *Latin Name – Common Name Index* 124

Suggested Reading 128

Chapter 1

The Ten Elements of Great Health

As a human being, you are a physical, mental, emotional and spiritual ecosystem....

It is important to understand that good physical health does not exist independently of our thoughts, feelings and beliefs, as well as the lifestyle decisions we make. We each exist in a personal and collective ecosystem where our physical bodies interrelate with our internal processes and our external surroundings. No system of health care, herbal or otherwise, can "cure" a physical condition existing in an ecosystem that is out of balance.

Personal choice is the most important element in maintaining the health of our ecosystem. Who we are is the sum of the choices that we make every day. We constantly choose what to think, what to eat and drink, who to be with, what to talk about, when to exercise, how much sleep to get, which movies to watch, and so forth. All of these choices may seem insignificant when we make them one by one. But when we add them together, they have a tremendous impact on our bodies. For example, occasionally going to a fast food restaurant does not have major health consequences. However when fast-foods become our main food supply, two things happen simultaneously. Our bodies become overloaded with fats, omega 6 fatty acids, sodium, free radicals, preservatives, food additives and many health-depleting substances. At the same time our bodies become starved for fiber, vitamins, minerals, omega 3 fatty acids, and other essential nutrients. Over a period of time, this type of diet leads to degenerative diseases. It may take time, but it will happen. The bottom line is that each choice we make is either health enhancing or health depleting.

Maintaining our ecosystem is a dynamic process. It is like being on a seesaw. As we move away from our center, our energy becomes increasingly out of balance and we are more subject to extreme highs and lows. Conversely,

The Ten Elements of Good Health

the sooner we take measures to stay close to our pivot point of balance, the less energy we need to expend to stay healthy. This additional energy can then be used for doing the things in our lives that give us joy, happiness, and contentment.

As a society, we have become overly dependent on doctors, drugs and surgery to maintain our health. Doctors have not been trained to inquire about and to recognize the neglect of the ten essential elements. Perhaps this is also why most people miss the point: the obvious is easy to overlook. By far, most of us get sick because we neglect to take care of the basics regularly. The good news is that optimal health is incredibly simple to attain and maintain. Take personal responsibility for your health and integrate these ten elements into your every day life.

If you wish to optimize your health and increase your resilience, or if you are confronted with health issues, I suggest you take a look at the following ten areas. What choices will you make today? Balance these ten elements on a daily basis and gain or maintain good health.

1. EXERCISE: Are you exercising regularly?
Exercise at least five times a week for one-half to three-quarters of an hour a day. One of the best forms of exercise is walking because it is low impact, aerobic, and inexpensive! The importance of exercise cannot be overestimated.

2. REST: Are you getting enough rest?
Set aside some time every day to relax, breathe and reconnect with yourself. Make it a priority to get enough restful sleep; sleep time before midnight is the most beneficial. Taking a short nap during the day is recommended.

3. NUTRITION: Is your diet fully supporting your body?
Eat whole foods and organic foods. Eat a variety of whole grains, vegetables and fruits. The more colorful the fruits and vegetables you eat, the better they are for you. Focus on the color purple, blue, red, yellow and green. Include at least one portion a day of the following green leafy vegetables: Swiss and red chard, kale, collards, Brussels

sprouts, parsley, mustard greens, turnip greens, chicory greens, dandelion greens, beet greens, spinach, cabbage, watercress, purslane, okra, and broccoli. Take a full-spectrum vitamin/mineral supplement every day to supplement your diet. Drink up to 1/2 ounce of water per pound of body weight a day to stay fully hydrated (the recommended ideal amount is about eight eight-ounce glasses a day). Don't forget to take your herbs!

4. NATURE: Do you spend enough time outdoors?

Nothing can replace being in nature when it comes to balancing your ecosystem. Devote time daily to get fresh air and sun. The good effects of adequate amounts of sunlight go beyond the production of vitamin D and emotional balance. It is easy to get your daily sun allowance when you take your regular walk during the day.

5. CREATIVITY: Do you have some sort of creative outlet that keeps you physically and mentally active?

Creative outlets can range from hobbies, gardening, writing, painting or other ways to express your inner self. Working in moderation in a field that you enjoy is also nurturing, self-affirming, and rewarding. Staying active and in contact with other individuals engaged in creative projects is integral to good health.

6. EMOTIONAL BALANCE: Are you emotionally healthy?

Choose to cultivate joy, love, gratitude and a sense of humor to nourish your ecosystem. Do you have repetitive episodes of anger, fear or grief that keep you out of balance? There is nothing wrong with having feelings. However, emotional imbalance becomes an issue when feelings are either repressed or allowed

Damiana

The Ten Elements of Good Health 15

to irrationally rule us. If either of these extremes is true for you, take measures to identify and change these negative emotional patterns.

7. GOALS: Do you have a sense of purpose?
To thrive, everyone should have something—whether it's doing volunteer work, spearheading a project, or working toward a goal—that demands mental activity. We all need direction and a sense of purpose in life. Goals give meaning to our lives. Giving back to our community through volunteering is life affirming.

8. MUTUAL SUPPORT: Are you giving and receiving love in your life?
Having a loving and accepting support system is critical to healing and staying healthy. Ecosystems, by their very nature, are dependent upon relationships. Giving and getting support and love from your family, friends or support group is essential to good health.

9. FAITH: Do you regularly communicate with your Higher Self or your Higher Power?
When we are connected to a higher power, it is much easier to feel balanced and fulfilled in life. Make time daily for this aspect of yourself. Ask for spiritual guidance from your higher power to help you in your daily life.

10. CHOICE: Do you take personal responsibility for your life?
Taking responsibility for your actions is a critical step in creating a healthy body, mind, soul and spirit. Of all the points presented, I believe that choice accounts for nearly half of our driving force for healing or staying healthy. At any given moment, you have many choices. Taking personal responsibility is the key that unlocks the door to integrating and balancing all of the other elements of healthy living discussed above. Remember that each and every positive choice you make daily gives you the power to shape your life!

16 CHAPTER 1

Making positive changes in your life

Start on the road to wellness today. Choose one of the preceding ten steps. Make the appropriate changes. Focus on and practice that step on a daily basis for three months. Three months is the amount of time it takes to create a new habit. Once the chosen step becomes an integral part of your life, move on to another step. As you begin to rebalance your personal ecosystem, your rewards will soon become apparent. You'll have more energy, enhance your health and feel better about yourself.

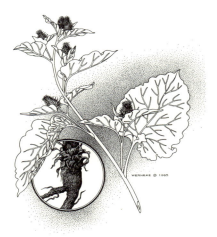

Burdock

CHAPTER 2

Understanding Herbal Medicine

Q: What is herbal medicine and who uses it?
Herbal medicine, sometimes called botanical medicine or phytotherapy, is the use of herbs for health purposes. Mankind has used herbs for millennia and thousands of herbs are recognized worldwide for their health benefits. According to the World Health Organization, 80 percent of the world's population still depends on herbal medicine as a primary form of healing. In the last 25 years, the United States has been experiencing a renaissance in the use of medicinal herbs. Traditional Chinese Medicine, Ayurvedic Medicine from India, Unani Tibb from Middle Eastern countries and South American herbs are becoming an integral part of the American herbal tradition.

Q: How does herbal medicine compare with current medical practices?
For some, herbal medicine is a total alternative to conventional allopathic medical treatments. For others, herbal medicine stands alongside conventional medicine as another choice, depending on the health issue at hand. Allopathic medicine aims at treating an illness or disease by inducing an opposite action in the body that suppresses the symptoms. Herbal medicine, on the other hand, aims at supporting the body in its efforts to heal itself, while addressing the cause.

Orthodox allopathic medicine is geared toward crisis management. Most individuals go to the doctor when their problems have escalated to the point that they require drastic measures, such as drugs or surgery. Drugs often have serious side effects and their costs can be prohibitive. In some instances the drugs given to patients are actually more dangerous than the diseases they are intended to treat. Surgery may eliminate the symptom but rarely addresses the cause. Drugs are often too strong and surgery too drastic for the problem at hand; however, in the orthodox medical system these are the major and, often, only treatment choices available. This is why people are turning to herbal medicine in growing numbers. It is geared toward prevention, is inexpensive, and has been shown to be safe and effective.

Herbal medicine assists the healing process by rebuilding and strengthening weak body systems, causing many persistent health problems to disappear. In the field of holistic medicine, herbs are not taken to "cure" disease but instead are used as tools to help rebalance and support the body in its quest for health.

Q: What healthcare benefits do herbs offer?

Herbs offer eight major healthcare benefits:

1. *Simplicity and accessibility:* Herbs are readily available to purchase in almost every conceivable delivery system, e.g.: capsules, tablets, tea bags, liquid herbal extracts, loose herbs, lozenges and salves. You can easily find these forms of herbs at your local natural products stores and natural pharmacies.

2. *Tolerance:* Many prescription drugs have adverse side effects that are often offset by additional drugs. Herbs, on the other hand, do not usually cause such a domino effect. They are generally easily absorbed and assimilated by the body and rarely cause side effects.

3. *Safety:* The bottom line is that herbs are inherently safe, but you must, as with any medications, respect and pay attention to dosage recommendations, contraindications, side effects or warnings.

4. *Effectiveness:* Many herbs, with their gentle actions, are usually not recognized by "experts" as having significant therapeutic benefits. However, anyone who has taken a cup of chamomile tea for sleep problems will attest to the fact that a noticeable relaxation follows its use. Additionally, since herbs do not contain just one single active principle, they cannot be "tested" in the same manner as drugs.

Understanding Herbal Medicine

However, thousands of years of herb usage have demonstrated that they are safe and effective healing agents.

5. Economy: Many herbs offer the same benefits as drugs for a fraction of what drugs cost. For example, Proscar ® costs a man suffering from benign prostatic hypertrophy (swollen prostate) approximately $3.00 a day for treatment. The same problem can be addressed with the herb Saw Palmetto for about 50 cents a day.

6. Empowerment: Herbs allow you, personally, do something for your health, at the precise time you need to do it.

7. Familiarity: Humans have ingested medicinal plants for thousands of years. Unlike drugs, herbs are not perceived by the body as foreign substances. They elicit a positive response from your body, helping it to return to a balanced state.

8. Environmental Friendliness: When herbs are certified organically grown or are ethically wildcrafted, their harvesting has very little or no negative impact on the planet. The pharmaceutical industry, on the other hand, manufactures drugs using complex and environmentally negative petroleum by-products and other chemicals.

Q: How do herbs differ from drugs?

There is a fundamental difference between how conventional drugs and herbs interact with the body. Conventional drugs work within the body for a limited time period and are designed to suppress the symptoms. Herbs, however, train the body for the future.

Antibiotics, frequently prescribed by conventional medical practitioners, bypass the immune system to kill

Oats

intruders; therefore, they do not teach the body how to defend itself in the future. Antibiotics create an ever-growing resistance among any remaining microorganisms and make them resistant to future rounds of antibiotics. Antibiotics also disrupt the ecology of the body and permit other negative microorganisms to grow and take over the normal flora in the intestines, as well as in other locations in the body. They also leave toxic residues that the body must either detoxify or store in its tissues.

On the other hand, herbs holistically help re-educate the body to heal itself. For example, *Echinacea* will stimulate your immune system not only to fight an infection, but also to recognize intruders a lot more rapidly and to respond more aggressively the next time your body encounters the same bug. Because commonly used medicinal herbs have little to no toxicity and leave no hard-to-deal-with residues, the body regains its balance more easily. None of the herbs addressed in this book leave negative residues in the body.

Metaphorically, drugs give a man a fish and feed him for a day. Herbs teach a man how to fish so that he can feed himself for a lifetime.

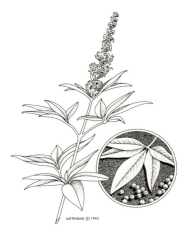

Vitex

Chapter 3

Choosing the Herbal Products that are Best for You

Q: In what forms are herbal products available?
The most popular herbal products in America are capsules and tablets. In the beverage category, herbal teas, especially in tea bags, account for a substantial amount of the herbs consumed in the United States. Bulk herbs are available in many herb, health and natural food stores. Liquid herbal extracts are also a popular way to ingest therapeutic herbal products. Each group has specific benefits and drawbacks.

Q: Which one of these forms offers the most therapeutic benefits?
Therapeutic benefits of herbs depend on a variety of factors. Is the herbal product fresh? Does it contain all of the active constituents in the ratios found in nature? Does the product have a long shelf life? Will the potency be intact when you are ready to take the product? Is a robust digestive system required to break down and deliver the plants' active constituents? Is the product convenient to take? Is it affordable? Does the product address the health issue that you are trying to resolve? Herbalists know that formulas in liquid herbal extract form affirmatively answer the above questions. This is the primary reason that a majority of American herbalists recommend and dispense liquid herbal extracts to their patients in their practice.

Q: What are liquid herbal extracts?
Liquid herbal extracts are herbs that have been processed so that their active constituents (ingredients) are suspended in a liquid medium, usually alcohol and water.

Q: Why do clinical herbalists prefer to recommend liquid herbal extracts?
Clinical herbalists prefer to recommend liquid herbal extracts for four reasons: freshness, potency, absorption, and formulation.

Freshness: Herbs in liquid herbal extract form retain their freshness and potency much longer than ground herbs in capsule or tablet form. Additionally, some herb parts, such as flowers, leaves and buds, are best processed while fresh (undried) to retain their full medicinal qualities. This critical step ensures that the essential oils and other fragile constituents found in them are not lost, evaporated or destroyed in the drying process.

These fresh herbs are picked from the field and shipped overnight in climate-controlled containers. Once released from quality control, the herbs are immediately ground to break the cell walls, added to an alcohol/water solution and extracted while fresh and vibrant. This process allows the release of their active constituents into the liquid solution. On the other hand, herbs sold in capsules, tablets, teas or as loose herbs, must first be dried and cannot deliver fresh (undried) herb benefits to the consumer.

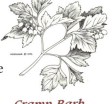

Cramp Bark

Conversely, there are situations where some herbs are best dried before being used. This is especially true with roots, barks, seeds and gums. The drying process deactivates certain enzymes and enhances the extraction and concentration of hardy glycosides, alkaloids and other stable active constituents. Grinding the herbs minutes before the extraction process using a super-cold (cryogenic) method with liquid nitrogen prevents the oxidation of the active constituents, evaporation of essential oils, and degradation of active constituents.

Potency: Herbalists have long recognized that potency is not about isolating a single "active ingredient" from an herb but results from the interaction of many constituents within each herb. Herbal products containing a full spectrum of bio-available constituents promote healing and the maintenance of health. Liquid herbal extracts consistently deliver more bioactive constituents than any other herbal supplements.

Choosing Herbal Products Best for You 23

Absorption: Experience has proven that liquid herbal extracts are the most effective delivery method for the body to absorb medicinal herbs. Since the active constituents are in a liquid solution, they bypass the digestive process and enter the bloodstream rapidly. Once assimilated, the herbs start working in the body within minutes.

Formulation: Clinical research shows that herbal formulas, a combination of several herbs, produce better results than single herbs. In a formula, each herb supports a specific body system in a manner that complements the action of the other herbs. Well-designed, time-tested formulations address the body's complete healing needs.

Q: Why are herbs in liquid herbal extract form preferable to dried herbs in capsule or tablet form?

The success of herbal products as healing agents is dependent on the availability and activity of their constituents when you ingest them. For maximum therapeutic benefits, therefore, it is very important to take herbs in the form that best captures and preserves these constituents. Liquid herbal extracts offer the most therapeutically beneficial form of herbs available on the market today.

Most herbs found in tablets or capsules are ground months prior to encapsulation. They lose many of their active constituents during the grinding process and while in storage. Herbal tablets also contain fillers, binders and other materials necessary to compress the ground herbs into tablet form. In addition, the body must dissolve tablets before it can begin to break down and assimilate the herbs.

Herbal capsules tend to be better than tablets because they do not contain the extra manufacturing materials and they dissolve easily in the stomach. However, herbs in capsules tend to oxidize more rapidly than those in tablets. Furthermore, when the digestive tract of a person is not functioning optimally, the potential therapeutic benefits of herbs in tablet and capsule form are decreased because the digestive system must free the active constituents from the fiber and cellulose. Herbs in liquid extract form, on the other hand, contain no fillers, binders, or "extra" ingredients, and keep their potency for a long time. They are immediately available for assimilation into the bloodstream, glands and organs. The extraction process removes the active constituents from the fresh or dried herbs and puts them into a solution that preserves them. Even a person with poor digestion can enjoy maximum benefits from liquid herbal extracts.

Q: What are the different kinds of liquid herbal extracts available?
Liquid herbal extracts are available in three basic forms, alcohol-containing extracts, non alcohol extracts and softgels. All three products should start as alcohol-containing extracts.

Q: How is each type of liquid herbal extract made?
Alcohol-containing extracts: Alcohol-containing liquid herbal extracts are produced by subjecting ground or powdered herbs, to individualized ratios of water and alcohol for specific lengths of time. This process captures the active constituents of these herbs. Fresh (undried) herbs are extracted using a kinetic maceration method. Using this method, herbs are first continuously agitated in an alcohol and water solution for 12 to 24 hours, and then soaked in that same liquid solution for a minimum of two weeks. For dried herbs, the active constituents are extracted in a special glass funnel called a "cold-extraction percolator." Using this method, an alcohol and water solution is poured over ground dried herbs in the cold-extraction percolator. Notice that, in both methods, no heat is ever used since heat damages the potency of the herbs' active principles.

Non alcohol extracts: To produce quality non alcohol liquid herbal extracts, the methods outlined above are used to extract the herbs and the totality of the active constituents in the alcohol and water mixture. Once the active constituents are in suspension, the next step consists of removing the alcohol using a low-heat vacuum

Choosing Herbal Products Best for You 25

process. The alcohol must be removed gently, without the use of heat, as heat negatively affects the potency of herbs. Then glycerine is added to the non alcohol extract as a carrier for the herbal constituents and to bring the extract back to its original volume. Finally, citric acid, a natural preservative found in citrus fruits, is added to prevent the growth of microorganisms in the extract.

Liquid herbal softgels: First, an alcohol-containing extract is made in the same way as described above. Then using a low-heat (room temperature) vacuum process the alcohol is removed. To this liquid concentrate, organic extra virgin olive oil is blended in. This concentrated extract is then encapsulated into a softgel. Each softgel contains the same amount of concentrated herbal extract as one dropperful of an alcohol-containing extract.

Regardless of the end product produced, there are three important steps that must be followed to create potent and effective liquid herbal extracts. First, all products must start as alcohol-containing extracts. This ensures that all of the active constituents are extracted out of the herbs. Second, no heat must ever be used at any point of the manufacturing process, as heat is very detrimental to the potency of herbal products. Third, it is essential that the full spectrum of active constituents be found in the final product. Only then can an herbal extract deliver on its healing promises.

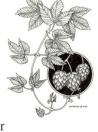

Hops

Q: Why are some liquid herbal extracts made with fresh herbs while others are made with dried herbs?

The reason herbalists use either fresh herbs or dried herbs in a formulation depends on the therapeutic objectives, i.e., why you are taking the herbs. Stinging Nettle, for example, can be used fresh or dried. To increase mineral absorption, dried Stinging Nettle offers the most benefits. On the other hand, fresh Stinging Nettle offers strong hay fever relief; once it is dried, its hay fever-alleviating properties virtually disappear. Other herbs, such as California Poppy, Oat Seed, Passionflower and Shepherd's Purse, should be processed while fresh in order to preserve their delicate volatile oils and other fragile constituents. Certain herbs, such as Blue Cohosh, Dong Quai, Goldenseal and Milk Thistle, are better used dried because the drying process modifies and enhances their medicinal action.

Whether you choose fresh herbs or dried herbs depends on each herb's specific constituents and the therapeutic goal you are trying to achieve. Therefore, some liquid herbal extracts and softgels are made from fresh herbs and others are made from dried herbs. In many formulas, fresh and dried forms are best blended together. This assures that you get the best form of each herb for the specific problems you are addressing.

Q: Why should liquid herbal extracts always start with an alcohol and water extraction?

There are three main reasons why alcohol and water are used to make quality liquid herbal extracts.

First, both alcohol and water are necessary to ensure full extraction of all the active constituents of the herbs. Goldenseal root best illustrates this principle. Boiling the root in water will quickly extract its water-soluble properties, of which the main one is called berberine. However, even boiling the roots for hours will fail to extract another constituent called hydrastine. Hydrastine, Goldenseal's main anti-inflammatory constituent, is only alcohol soluble. It takes a minimum of 70 percent alcohol to extract it from Goldenseal roots. Using a liquid that contains the proper ratio of water and alcohol is the best way to get all of the constituents out of each herb.

Second, alcohol assists in the proper absorption of the herb by your digestive tract.

Third, alcohol acts as a natural preservative, preventing microbial contamination and assuring a long shelf life.

Choosing Herbal Products Best for You 27

The alcohol content in different extracts ranges from as little as 20 percent to as high as 95 percent. The amount of alcohol required for maximum extraction is dependent upon the properties of each and every herb. Note that vinegar and glycerine cannot replace alcohol as efficient extractive agents.

Q: The label of an herbal extract says it contains 70 percent alcohol. Does that mean the remaining 30 percent is water? What percentage of the mixture are herbs?

If an herbal extract label states that it contains 70 percent alcohol, the other parts of the liquid may be water and/or glycerine. However, 100 percent of the mixture in the bottle contains herbs. To illustrate this point, let's use an analogy. Let's say you start with four ounces of water. Add one ounce of sugar into the four ounces of water. Interestingly, you still only have four ounces of water, but the water is now sweet and permeated with sugar. The sugar is contained within the water but is no longer visible as a separate ingredient. The same concept applies to herbal extracts. If a particular extract contains a liquid made of 70 percent alcohol and 30 percent water, both the alcohol and the water are imbued with herbs. The liquid holds the herbal constituents in suspension just as the water in the analogy holds the sugar.

Q: How much alcohol will I ingest when I take an average dose of an alcohol-containing liquid herbal extract?

Although some people may be concerned about the amount of alcohol in alcohol-containing liquid herbal extracts, there is little cause for worry. On average, 30 drops of a liquid herbal extract containing 70 percent alcohol (see the label on the bottle for the actual percentage of alcohol found in the product) contains about the same amount of alcohol as one ripe banana. In addition, when a person eats fruit, the body ferments it in the digestive tract, producing alcohol. The point I am emphasizing here is that most alcohol-sensitive people do not quit eating fruits because the fermentation within their gastrointestinal tract produces alcohol. The liver is the organ responsible for the processing and breakdown of any alcohol produced by digestive fermentation or ingested through herbal extracts.

Q: A ripe banana's worth of alcohol is still too much for me. How can I reduce the amount of alcohol in a dosage and still get the maximum benefits of a liquid herbal extract?

Evaporating the alcohol out of an alcohol-containing liquid herbal extract is best done on a dose-by-dose basis. Do not heat an entire bottle of extract as the amount of heat required to evaporate the alcohol would damage the herbs in the extract. Instead, add the number of drops of the extract to a cup of boiling water, or, if you wish, to an herbal tea that is naturally caffeine-free. Let the mixture sit for 5-10 minutes. Forty to sixty percent of the alcohol will evaporate during that time. In an extract containing 70 percent alcohol, the remaining alcohol after evaporation will be about the same as you would find in a third of a ripe banana. Evaporating the alcohol on a dose-by-dose basis does not in any way diminish the effectiveness of the herbs, because the heat is not sustained and does not adversely affect the active constituents.

Q: Some of the forumulations presented in this book have oats. Are oats gluten-free and are they safe for celiac disease patients?

In the last few years, gluten-free products have gained favor with the public. However, for celiac disease patients and other gluten-sensitive individuals, the purity of gluten-free products (and sometimes the lack thereof) is a critical element that may adversely affect their health.

Six products reviewed in this book contain oat (*Avena sativa*). These products include Deep Sleep®, Deprezac™, Kava Cool Complex™, Nervine Tonic™, Smoke Free®, and Stress *ReLeaf*®. The oat seeds used in these formulations are harvested while fresh and in the milky stage; this is the stage just before the grain becomes fully formed. At that growth stage, a white, milky liquid is released when the seed is crushed. It is at this precise stage that the oat seed delivers the most benefits to the nervous system.

Choosing Herbal Products Best for You

The reason celiac disease individuals seem to react to oats is not that oats contain gluten but that the oats they eat are contaminated by wheat, barley or rye gluten. A study conducted by a scientist in 2008 showed that of the 109 oat food samples obtained from Europe, the United States and Canada, the majority were highly contaminated with wheat, barley, rye, or a mixture of these three cereals. These elevated gluten levels from contaminated oats would create problems in celiac disease patients.

Some have argued that, in large quantities, oats may cause a reaction in celiac disease patients. However, recent clinical studies have demonstrated that celiac patients can safely include clean oats in a gluten-free diet. Scientific research clearly shows that clean oats do not contribute to adverse effects in individuals suffering from celiac disease. Cross-contamination with gluten-containing grains is the greater concern for these individuals.

Oats contamination with wheat, rye, barley, and spelt may occur when these seeds are inadvertently mixed up with oats and are then planted in the fields. Contamination can also occur during the harvesting, cleaning, storing, milling, and food processing of oats. Keeping the oat grains away from the gluten-containing grains is essential. Good agricultural and manufacturing practices must be in place and maintained on farms as well as in the food/herbal supplement industry. It's also important that the use of harvesting, cleaning, or milling equipment as well the use of storage containers or silos be dedicated to oats only.

Here are four steps manufacturers should follow to ensure that the oat products you purchase are gluten-free.

1. Ensure that the farmers who grow their oats do not grow wheat, barley, rye or spelt in their fields. This step guarantees that cross-contamination occurrences are non-existent.

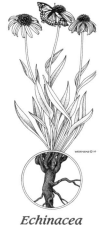

Echinacea angustifolia

2. Ensure that the chain of custody is well controlled from the farm to the finished product. That means that the manufacturer must know every step that occurs from the time the oats are sown, harvested, and shipped to the manufacturing facility. The chain of custody must include the processing of oats into the final herbal product.

3. Ensure that the equipment used to harvest, clean, mill, process or store the oats should be dedicated to that grain only and not shared with any other gluten-containing grains

4. Perform analytical testing on the oat extracts and the finished products, preferably using the state-of-the-art Elisa® method to ensure that the gluten levels are lower than 20 parts per million (20 ppm).

The most important point to remember is that oats are safe for celiac disease patients AS LONG AS the oats are clean and free of other offending grains like wheat, barley and rye.

Q: I am a recovering alcoholic or I need to avoid alcohol as part of my religious beliefs. What are my herbal options for a strong, effective herbal product?

Even though the alcohol left in the product is very low after evaporation, in my opinion, you should honor and protect your recovery or your religious beliefs and stay away from any alcohol-containing products. I suggest that you seek non alcohol extracts, liquid herbal softgels or other forms of herbs that are in a non-alcoholic form.

Q: I have read that I should buy herbs that are "standardized". What is standardization?

Standardization of herbal products occurs when a specific amount of one "active constituent" in an herb is brought to a specific level. For example, Valerian is available in a standardized two percent valerenic acid form.

In the last two decades there has been a strong push by a segment of the herbal industry to "standardize" herbal products. This phenomenon is occurring principally because of two strong influences. First, medical doctors are being introduced to herbs by patients who are increasingly uncomfortable with prescription

Choosing Herbal Products Best for You

drugs and who are requesting products with fewer side effects and made from more natural sources. Second, coming from an orthodox, pharmaceutically-driven framework, medical doctors have been conditioned through their training to recommend products that have "active ingredients" in measurable and consistent amounts. Thus, they are encouraging the trend to standardize herbs. In response to pressure from medical doctors, standardized herbal products, some herb companies are developing and marketing products.

However, the problem with standardizing herbal products becomes apparent when one looks at all the constituents found in an herb. A person quickly realizes that it is nearly impossible to answer the question, "Which of the numerous constituents found in an herb should be designated as being the effective one?" A quick overview of the attempts to standardize Valerian root reveals some of the problems inherent with this approach. A few decades ago, it was thought that essential oils were the active constituents of Valerian. But when the isolated essential oils were administered to patients, the results were less than satisfactory. Later, it was thought that valepotriates were the active ingredients until research demonstrated only marginal results. Still later, valerenic acid was thought to be the active ingredient. More clinical research, same unsatisfactory results. The irony is that each round of testing actually support the fact that whole Valerian root give better results than any of the "standardized" fractions of the herb.

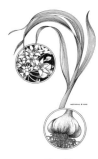

Garlic

In my opinion, standardization runs counter to the holistic view that each herb is an ecosystem where all of its parts heal and balance our bodies. Additionally, in Germany, many nutraceutical companies have recognized this fact and are now producing herbal medicine formulations that emphasize whole herb extracts instead of standardized fractions.

Q: Does standardization increase the healing potential of herbs?

Considerable debate on this subject exists. I strongly believe that, in most instances, using whole herbs is superior to standardizing herbal fractions. In support to this point of view, I point to three issues that are unresolved in the debate of this topic.

First, in over 98 percent of the herbs available in the marketplace, it is virtually unknown what the active constituents might be. For example, in the preceding Q&A, Valerian root clearly illustrates that the question, "Which one of the many constituents found in the herb is the "active ingredient"? is still unanswered. Here's another interesting example. In the late 1970s and the early 1980s, researchers thought that the polysaccharides in *Echinacea* possessed the entire immunostimulating activities of the herb. Based on this research, some European companies standardized their *Echinacea* products to achieve a specific amount of polysaccharides (usually labeled as echinacosides). However, subsequent research revealed that alcohol-soluble constituents were even more effective in supporting the immune system than the polysaccharides. Additionally, every year, new *Echinacea* compounds are isolated and identified.

The second issue is that the standardization of a few effective products has been assumed to be possible for all herbs. Certainly, there are a handful of standardized herbal products that have been shown to be effective in specific situations. For instance, Milk Thistle with standardized silymarin levels is used for serious

Choosing Herbal Products Best for You

liver diseases, while Bilberry's anthocyanins have been shown to support healthy vision. However, if you are using Milk Thistle to protect your liver, a formula containing whole-seed liquid extract protects the liver just as well as a standardized extract, at a fraction of the cost. Many of the constituents that protect the liver are present in whole Milk Thistle seed extract but are absent from standardized Milk Thistle product. Additionally, whole Bilberry and Blueberry deliver not only anthocyanins but a multitude of other compounds that support our bodies. The point is that the successful standardization of about a half dozen herbs (Bilberry, Ginkgo, Grape Seed extract, Gugulipid, Kava, Milk Thistle and Saw Palmetto) is simply not applicable to all herbs. Remember that in over 98 percent of herbs, we simply do not know what the "active" ingredients are.

Finally, the debate and practice of standardizing herbs is another instance where science tries to improve Nature by dissecting her. Research in the standardization of Feverfew provides a pertinent example. For years, it was thought that parthenolides were the active constituents of Feverfew. Many Feverfew products from the 1980s and 1990s were standardized to contain a minimum amount of parthenolides. However, the latest research has shown that even when parthenolides are removed from Feverfew extract, people suffering from migraine headaches continue to get good results from its use. The question, then, "What is the active ingredient of herb x?" remains to be solved for

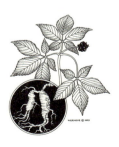

American Ginseng

most herbs. In my opinion, science has failed to prove that standardized products are superior to whole herb extracts for the vast majority of herbs.

Q: What is the shelf life of herbs in different forms?

Form	Shelf Life
Powdered herbs (roots and leaves)	1-6 months
Tea bags	3-12 months
Herbal capsules	3-12 months
Whole dried leaves	12 months
Herbal tablets	3-24 months
Whole dried roots	1-3 years
Alcohol-free liquid extracts	5 years
Liquid herbal extract in softgels	5 years
Alcohol-containing liquid extracts	5-20 years or more

This chart points out that the more an herb is reduced in size, the more herb surface area is exposed and the more rapidly it loses its beneficial properties. In general, whole herbs retain their medicinal properties or "shelf life" longer than ground herbs. Roots, barks, seeds and gums tend to retain their potency longer than herbs, flowers, leaves and buds. This chart also shows that liquid herbal extracts maintain the longest shelf life of all other forms of herbs. In fact, I have liquid herbal extracts that I have made more than 30 years ago that are still very potent. Once the herbs are extracted in a liquid medium, very little oxidation or degradation of active constituents occurs.

Q: How should I care for liquid herbal extracts to keep them fresh?

For optimum shelf life, I suggest a three-point approach. First, keep your extracts away from direct sunlight as well as away from windows or other sources of light. Second, keep your extracts away from hot temperatures (e.g., do not keep them in your car in the summertime.) Third, keep bottle caps firmly closed. With alcohol-containing extracts, no refrigeration is ever required. However, I believe it is a good idea to refrigerate non

Choosing Herbal Products Best for You

alcohol extracts once they are opened.

Q: How can I tell if an extract has "gone bad"?
In my experience with alcohol-containing liquid herbal extracts, it is rare for extracts not to last for years when they are stored properly. When purchasing non alcohol liquid herbal extracts, always look for a product that contains citric acid, a natural preservative. Should the product lack a preservative such as citric acid, smell the extract. If the product has a musty odor or seems to have something growing in it, discard it. Even with a citric acid-containing, alcohol-free product, refrigerate the extract once it is opened and discard within six months of opening.

Q: Does it matter if the herbs I take are from an organic source?
As a clinical herbalist concerned about our environment, I strongly recommend that herbal consumers choose organically grown herbs.

First, choosing organically cultivated herbs helps lessen the over-harvesting of herbs in the wild. Second, certified organic farmers make sure they have crops year after year by not compromising their land for short-term gain. Therefore, by buying organic, you support a constant renewal of our herbal medicine supplies. Third, certified organic farmers are inspected by a third-party certifying agency, making certain that farmers practice sustainable, chemical-free and pesticide-free farming techniques. This ensures that the herbs you buy support not only your individual healing but also support the health of our planet.

Q: What should I look for when I buy liquid herbal extracts or liquid herbal softgels?
Sufficient Alcohol Content: Choose alcohol-containing extracts that contain a minimum of 20 percent alcohol to act as a preservative and to prevent contamination by fungus and bacteria. Additionally, alcohol levels higher than 20 percent are needed to extract most herbs. For example, Milk Thistle and Cayenne need at least 95 percent alcohol in order to extract all of the active constituents. *Echinacea* and Goldenseal require 70 percent alcohol to extract their constituents,

while herbs like Peppermint and Chamomile require a much lower alcohol percentage.

Properly Made Non Alcohol Extracts: When selecting an non alcohol extract, choose one that has been extracted with alcohol and that had the alcohol removed using a gentle, low-heat process. This way, you will get all the benefits of the alcohol-containing extracts minus the alcohol. Citric acid should be added to non alcohol extracts as a natural preservative.

Properly Made Liquid Herbal Softgels: When selecting a liquid herbal softgel, choose one where the herbs were first extracted with alcohol and where the alcohol was gently removed, using a low-heat process. Choose softgels that contain extra virgin olive oil, because of its low oxidation capacity as compared to other types of oils.

Cold Processing: When extracts are made from whole herbs ground cryogenically (cold grinding) minutes prior to extraction, no constituents are destroyed during the grinding process by friction-induced heat. Cold-process kinetic maceration for fresh herbs or cold-process percolation for dried herbs yields more active constituents in the finished extracts than in herbs processed using other methods.

Organically Grown Herbs: Choose herbal extracts made from certified organically grown herbs when possible. When certified organically grown herbs are not available, choose products made from wild-harvested herbs picked in regions that are not exposed to pesticides, herbicides, or chemical fertilizers. Additionally look for a manufacturer who is a certified organic processor.

Liquid Herbal Extract Formulations: Whenever possible choose herbal formulas. They offer more benefits than single herbs. The formulas listed in this book have been blended, tested and approved by Medical Herbalist Daniel Gagnon.

Chapter 4

Taking Herbal Medicine Extracts

Q: Why are herbal formulas a better choice than single herbs?

To address your health concerns, it is important to choose the herbs that best address your specific condition. This book lists both single herbal extracts and formulas as effective healing agents. However, I generally favor formulas because they offer you greater health benefits, greater affordability and greater convenience.

For example, if you look in books or on Internet sites under the heading of arthritis, you'll see a plethora of single herbs recommended for that purpose. These may include Alfalfa, Angelica, Black Cohosh, Boswellia, Devil's Claw and many others. You read the description for each herb and try to figure out if this is the herb for you. Ultimately, my patients admit that they are confused about which herbs to take for their health challenges. A considerable amount of knowledge of the body's functions and of your particular symptoms is required to choose the most appropriate herbs for each condition.

On the other hand, when you read the description of the formula Arthrotonic™, you will see that it combines Devil's Claw and nine other herbs, which all perform specific functions to relieve the symptoms of arthritis and help the body get healthy again. The formula Loviral™ contains Lomatium, Pelargonium (umckaloabo) and Osha roots, among many other herbs, all of which address respiratory viral infections. With herbal formulas, the guesswork of determining which single extracts to take to address your specific health issue is eliminated. Additionally, the cost of buying one or two formulas versus buying all of the single extracts included in each formula is significantly less. The level of support, in this case, for your arthritis or viral infection, is greatly amplified because each formula is stronger than the sum of its individual herbal parts. Each herb complements the others and together they act in a synergistic way to strengthen and support your body in its quest for health.

Q: Do I use herbs differently when I have an acute condition, as opposed to when I have a chronic condition?

Absolutely. During an **acute phase** (rapid onset, severe symptoms, and quick resolution, as in colds or flu) of a condition, it is desirable to take herbs on a frequent basis to maintain a consistently high level of the herbs' active constituents in the bloodstream. This way, the stimulation, sedation, or balancing that the herbs offer are constantly bathing the affected tissues. However, should the therapeutic level in the bloodstream of the herbs fall, the invading microorganisms or the inflammation threatening the tissues will continue to rise. Your body must then redouble in its efforts to get the affected tissues back to normal. Taking care of an acute phase quickly and completely prevents the problem from becoming chronic or recurrent.

During a **chronic phase** (long duration, ongoing or recurring symptoms) of a disease it is important to take herbs on a regular basis over a longer period of time in order to offer the challenged tissues the healing support they need. In this phase, you need to supply tissues with nutrients and herbal substances on a daily basis so that the tissues can heal and resume their normal healthy functions.

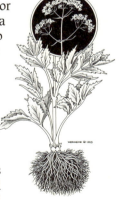

Valerian

Arthritis again provides us with a clear example of how herbs address acute versus chronic phases of a health condition. In the chronic phase of arthritis, a person will have stiffness and dull pain in the joints; whereas during an acute flare-up, inflammation, sharper pain, as well as swelling, will be present. Both phases should be addressed, but in different ways. In an acute arthritis flare-up, the strategy is to decrease inflammation and get rid of the waste products that are contributing to the inflammation. This requires frequent dosages. During a chronic arthritic phase, the strategy is to stabilize and help repair the tissues, and prevent future flare-ups. This requires larger dosages, taken fewer times a day, over longer periods of time.

Q: What is the best time of day to take liquid herbal extracts?

Ideally, I suggest taking extracts between meals, apart from food, when it is the easiest for the body to absorb them. By taking them on an empty stomach, the extracts are not competing with food for absorption and enter the bloodstream rapidly and immediately start the healing process. A few herbs, however, are better taken before meals. For example, bitter herbs help to tone the digestive function and improve production of hydrochloric acid and other digestive enzymes. Others, like sleep aid herbs, are better taken one hour before bedtime to promote relaxation and restful sleep. Note the suggested use under each herb in the Herbal Directory section (Chapter 7) for specific directions on timing.

Q: How do I know when it's time to stop taking an extract?

Some herbs act very quickly, while others need more time to balance, nourish and support body systems. Certain herbs are best taken for a short time (one to three weeks) while other herbs yield their best results when they are taken for longer periods (one to six months or longer). When duration is specifically important, it will be noted in the suggested use section in the Herbal Directory section (Chapter 7).

The following types of considerations determine duration. In general, the stronger the herb, the shorter the length of time it should be taken. Examples of some stronger herbs include Goldenseal and Lomatium. Other herbs, such as **Ginkgo, Hawthorn, Oat Seed and St. John's Wort, must be taken for a minimum of one month** before they begin to positively affect the physiology with their healing qualities. Therefore, those herbs should be taken for several months in order to achieve best results.

Formulas designed to be taken for acute conditions, such as Peak Defense™ for colds and flu, should be taken for shorter amounts of time. On the other hand, formulas aimed at chronic problems, such as Deprezac™ for depression, and formulas taken as long-term tonic, such as, Deep Health® as a deep immune system tonic, require longer periods of ingestion, as their benefits accumulate over time. If duration is not indicated, then take the herb until symptoms cease. If you are in doubt, consult a knowledgeable herbalist, a naturopath or herbal-savvy primary care physician. Keep in mind that herbs are medicine and recommended dosages should not be exceeded.

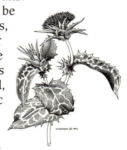

Milk Thistle

Q: Since I am dealing with several different health problems, what is the best way to take herbs in this situation?

When taking different herbs for different health problems, there are four points to keep in mind. These guidelines are applicable to all age groups.

1. Aim for the root cause of your problems rather than just treating separate symptoms. For example, a person may experience difficulty sleeping, sour stomach, cystitis, sinusitis, and nervousness. If each symptom is treated as a separate problem, herbs will be needed for the urinary, digestive and respiratory systems, as well as for the nervous system. But in this case, the individual may simply need herbs targeting stress. Conversely, the digestive system may need support. Interestingly, when the root cause is addressed with the appropriate formula, seemingly unrelated symptoms disappear without even addressing them directly.

2. Take herbs for different problems at different times. Take herbs for the same problem at the same time. For example, if you want to take Arthrotonic™ for arthritis and Migra-Free® to prevent migraine headaches, I suggest you take them about 15 minutes apart. On the other hand, if you are taking different herbs for the same problem, such as Immune Alert™ and Congest Free™ for a cold, the extracts can be combined and taken at the same time.

3. Ideally, take different herbal formulas at least fifteen minutes apart. Conversely, if taking the herbs fifteen minutes apart means that you will forget to take the next dosage or simply skip it, then it would be better to take the dosages together.

4. Address no more than three health issues at once. Let's say you are taking herbs for asthma, arthritis and migraines, but you also suffer from skin rashes and chronic fatigue. Decide which three conditions to address by aiming for the root causes of the problems. Most often the longest-standing problems are the ones to address first.

Q: Can I take herbal extracts at the same time I am taking conventional drugs?

Yes, in many instances taking herbs at the same time as conventional drugs will actually support and heal the body faster and more thoroughly. For example, taking immune stimulating herbs while you are on antibiotics is recommended, because these herbs will strengthen the immune system and prevent relapses after the round of antibiotics is completed.

Q: Some liquid herbal extracts taste fairly bitter. What are the benefits of bitter tastes?

Don't let taste keep you from enjoying the healing benefits of herbs. It is interesting to note that in our society, we are addicted to two basic tastes: salty and sweet. But there are three other tastes that are equally important in maintaining health: sour, bitter, and pungent. These tastes, when taken as herbs or foods, initiate body reactions that help restore and maintain health. For example bitter herbs, such as Gentian, help support the digestive functions. On the other hand, pungent tasting herbs, such as Turmeric, help tone the liver. It is important to remember that herbs, even though they may not taste pleasant, nevertheless put us in touch with Nature's pure energy to assist us in our quest for health. However, if the taste of the herbs will prevent you from taking them, consider using liquid extracts in softgels.

Q: What is the best way to disguise the taste of liquid herbal extracts?

The best way to take alcohol-containing or non alcohol liquid herbal extracts without affecting their healing properties is to put them in eight ounces of water, juice, and/or herbal tea, as long as the tea is caffeine-free. Although some people choose to put undiluted liquid herbal extracts directly in their mouths, putting liquid extracts in a beverage of some type is preferable for most people. The easiest way to completely eliminate the taste of strong-tasting liquid herbal extracts is to take them as a softgel so they bypass the taste buds. However, herbs taken for digestion are best taken as a liquid herbal extract in two or three ounces of water. It is their bitter taste that supports and enhances digestive functions.

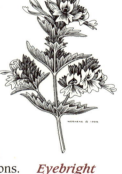

Eyebright

Q: Can I give liquid herbal extracts to my children?

Liquid herbal extracts are a convenient way to give herbs to children. However, there are five suggestions that you should be aware of.

1. Children should be at least one year old before being given herbs. For children under a year old, you should give extracts only under the supervision of an herbalist or knowledgeable primary care physician (medical doctor,

Taking Herbal Medicine Extracts 43

naturopath, acupuncturist, etc.). There are a few exceptions where mild herbs like lavender or chamomile can be given to infants.

2. A child's dosage is a fraction of the adult dosage. The rule of thumb is to take the smallest adult dose suggested and adjust it by giving one tenth the amount per year of age. For example, if an extract calls for a 20-drop dose for an adult, adjust the dosage by giving two drops per year of age to a child. In this example, a three-year-old child would take six drops of the extract (20 drops divided by 10 = 2 drops multiplied by the age of the child [3 years old] = 6 drops). If the extract called for a 30-drop dose for an adult, a four-year-old child would take 12 drops of the extract (30 drops divided by 10 = 3 drops times the age of the child [4 years old] = 12 drops).

3. Adjust the dosage for the individual child. If the child is of slight build or is underweight for his/her age, cut the suggested child's dosage by 25 percent.

4. If the child has a weak constitution, i.e.; is frail, recuperating from an illness, or is in a weakened state, cut the usual child's dosage by 25-50 percent. You can gauge and perhaps increase the dosage according to the child's response.

5. Clark's rule is a more accurate, though more burdensome, way to calculate a child's dosage. Clark's rule refers to a procedure used to calculate the amount of medicine to give to a child between the ages of 2 to 17. Divide the adult dosage by 150 pounds and multiply the answer by the weight of the child. For example, if the adult dosage is 30 drops and the child weighs 40 pounds, divide the amount (30 drops) by 150 pounds = 2/10 of a drop, and multiply it by the weight of the child (40 pounds) = 8 drops. Thus the child's dose in this case would be 8 drops.

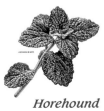

Horehound

Q: How can I get my child to take liquid herbal extracts?

Putting the drops in orange juice is the easiest way to give an herbal extract to a child, as orange juice best disguises the taste. Other juices may also do the trick. Additionally, non alcohol liquid herbal extracts have a pleasant citrus flavor and a sweet taste.

Q: Can I give liquid herbal extracts to my pets? How much should I give them?

I have found over the years that pets respond favorably to liquid herbal extracts. However, in the same way that you need to adjust dosages for children, care should be taken to adjust the dosage for animals. Use Clark's rule described above to adjust the dosage for the animal. Generally, the best way to give extracts to pets is to mix it in their food. It is not necessary to evaporate the alcohol, as the amount of alcohol in a dose is too small to harm them. Side Note- most pet owners use cheese, hot dogs or Pill Pockets® to adminster tablets, capsules, or softgels to cats and dogs.

Q: Can I compare powdered herbal capsules to liquid herbal extracts or softgels?

It is difficult to compare powdered herbal capsules to liquid herbal extracts especially when it comes to issues of potency. With herbal capsules, the body must first break down the plant fibers and then digest and assimilate the plant constituents. If a person taking herbal capsules or tablets has digestive problems, the break down and assimilation of the herbs will be incomplete. However, in the case of liquid extracts or softgels, because the constituents are already in solution, the body assimilates them rapidly and thoroughly.

When it comes to potency, herbal capsules contain ground herbs and lose potency through evaporation, oxidation and degradation, both during the manufacturing process and every day they sit on a shelf. Herbal capsules have a maximum of a one-year shelf life. On the other hand, because liquid herbal extracts are processed from fresh herbs or freshly ground dried herbs, their active constituents are preserved for a much longer period of time. Liquid herbal extracts or softgels keep their potency for a minimum of three years. Each liquid softgel offers the same benefits as taking a minimum of two capsules of ground herbs.

As mentioned earlier, perhaps the single most enticing benefit of using liquid herbal extracts and softgels made from liquid herbal extracts is that they can be made with fresh (undried) herbs. Some herbs contain constituents that are found only when the herb is fresh. California Poppy herb, Lemon Balm herb, Oat seed in the milky stage, Stinging Nettle leaf, and Valerian root are some examples of herbs that offer specific benefits in the fresh state that are not available to the user once the herb is dried.

Q: How can I compare the strength of herbal capsules to liquid herbal extracts?

Consult the following list to compare the approximate equivalencies of milligrams of dried herbs in capsule drops found in liquid herbal extracts and softgels. Keep in mind that liquid herbal extracts or liquid herbal softgels contain either extracts made from fresh (undried) herbs or made from freshly ground dried herbs while herbal capsules can only be made with pre-ground dried herbs.

1 drop = 25 mg of ground herbs in a capsule
2 drops = 50 mg of ground herbs in a capsule
20 drops = 500 mg of ground herbs in a capsule
One dropperful of extract = approximately 30 drops
One-ounce bottle of liquid herbal extract = approximately 1,200 drops
One-ounce bottle of liquid herbal extract = approximately 40 dropperfuls
Each one-ounce bottle of liquid herbal extract = approximately 60 capsules each containing 500 mg of ground herbs
One softgel = 30 drops = 500 mg of ground herbs in a regular capsule
60 softgels = approximately 120 regular capsules, each containing 500 mg of ground herbs.

Chapter 5

Deciding When to Avoid Certain Herbs

An informed consumer can exercise educated choices. This section is aimed at providing additional information to support the safe use of herbs.

Q: I am pregnant or nursing. What precautions should I use when taking herbs?
Some herbs should be avoided during pregnancy and nursing unless specifically recommended by a knowledgeable herbalist, naturopath or other primary care physician. Note and follow the recommendations and contraindications listed with each herb in the Herbal Directory (Chapter 7).

Herbs and Herbal Formulas to Avoid during Pregnancy

Adrenotonic™
Congest Free™
CranBladder *ReLeaf*®
Deprezac™
Essiac Tonic
HB Pressure™ Tonic
Herbaprofen®
Kava Cool Complex™
Kidney Tonic™
Liver Tonic™
Loviral™
Lymphatonic™
Menopautonic™
Nervine Tonic™
Osha Root Throat Syrup
ParaFree™
Peak Defense™
Phytocillin®
Respiratonic®
Smoke Free®
Stomach Tonic™
Stress *ReLeaf*®
Ultimate Ginseng™
Vibrant Energy™
Yeast *ReLeaf*®

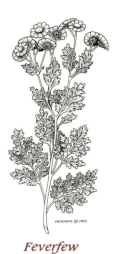

Feverfew

Deciding When to Avoid Certain Herbs

Herbs and Herbal Formulas to Avoid While Nursing

Congest Free™
Deprezac™
Herbaprofen®
Kava Cool Complex™
ParaFree™
Smoke Free®

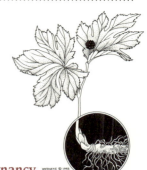

Goldenseal

Q: Besides during pregnancy and nursing, are there precautions for people who are taking prescription drugs or over-the-counter medication, or who belong to a specific age group should follow?

Yes, there are two points to keep in mind. First herbs can potentiate the action of prescription medications. Second, monitor the effects of herbs when given to the elderly or to very young children.

1. If you are taking conventional medication for a health problem, be aware that taking herbs that work on the same medical condition may increase the effect of the drugs. For example, if you are on medication for hypertension and start taking herbs to lower your blood pressure, your blood pressure may become abnormally low. Always monitor the results of taking any medications and herbs for specific medical conditions with your doctor and/or a person knowledgeable about the use of herbs and pharmaceuticals.

2. For children, especially those under the age of five, and also for adults over the age of 70, special care should be taken when administering herbs. Children and the elderly may be susceptible either to diarrhea or to overstimulation from certain herbs. Therefore it is important to start with smaller dosages and to monitor the reaction of the person. You will find that in most instances everything will be normal. But in a few cases, diarrhea, digestive upset, skin rash or other symptoms may occur, indicating the need to decrease the dosage or to stop giving herbs altogether.

Q: What are "contraindications"?

The word "contraindication" is defined by Taber's Cyclopedic Medical Dictionary (2005) as "any symptom or circumstance indicating the inappropriateness of a form of treatment otherwise advisable." When you choose herbs or herbals formulas for your health issues, consult the Herbal Directory (Chapter 7), and pay strict attention to the situations or conditions for which the herbs are contraindicated. Be sure to follow all the directions given with each herb or formula.

Q: What is a "side effect"? Do herbs have side effects like drugs?

Taber's Cyclopedic Medical Dictionary (2005) defines a side effect as "the action or effect, usually of a drug, other than that desired." In some instances an herb may simply have an effect that you should be aware of. For example, some herbs may change the color or smell of the urine. It is rare that an herb has negative drug-like side effects. This is one primary reason that so many people are turning to herbs as their preferred mode of treatment.

However, there are a few herbs listed in this book that may cause side effects if taken in larger amounts than recommended. In addition, there is always the possibility that a few individuals may have unpredictable reactions to herbs. Pay close attention to the suggested use and all applicable comments regarding contraindications and side effects in the Herbal Directory (Chapter 7). If you experience a disturbing side effect, discontinue use.

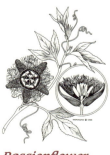

Passionflower

Deciding When to Avoid Certain Herbs 49

Q: What are "warnings for herbs"?
Webster's Encyclopedic Unabridged Dictionary defines warning as "serving to give notice, advice or intimation to a person of danger, possible harm or anything else unfavorable." A few of the herbs and herbal formulas listed in this book may cause undesirable outcomes or may interact with over-the-counter medications or prescription drugs in a negative way. Pay close attention to the suggested use and all applicable notations regarding contraindications in the Herbal Directory (Chapter 7).

The following three lists summarize contraindications, possible side effects and warning regarding herbs and herbal formulas found in this book.

Contraindications of Herbs:

Deprezac™—do not use with HIV protease inhibitors, cyclosporine, warfarin, and digoxin
Kava Cool Complex™—do not use with alcohol or barbiturates

Possible Side Effects of Herbs:

ChlorOxygen® Chlorophyll Concentrate—dark green stools may occur
CranBladder *ReLeaf*®—peculiar urine smell and color may occur
HB Pressure™ Tonic—may cause low blood pressure
Kava Cool Complex™—large amount over an extended period of time may cause skin rash
Kidney Tonic™—peculiar urine smell and color may occur
Loviral™—may cause skin rash
Smoke Free®—large doses of the extract may cause nausea

Warnings for Herbs:

Bug Itch *ReLeaf*® —for external use only
Deprezac™—do not use in bipolar syndrome and/or for any other severe depressive states; consult your primary care physician if you are taking other medications

DermaCillin™—for external use only. Product may cause a mild burning sensation when applied to broken skin. Discontinue use and consult with a doctor if condition worsens

HB Pressure™ Tonic—monitor your blood pressure to ensure a healthy blood pressure

Ivy Itch ReLeaf®—for external use only. Discontinue use and consult with a doctor if condition persists, worsens, or an infection occurs

Kava Cool Complex™—caution: US FDA advises that a potential risk of rare, but severe, liver injury may be associated with kava-containing dietary supplements. Ask a healthcare professional before use if you have or have had liver problems, frequently use alcoholic beverages, or are taking any medication. Stop use and see a doctor if you develop symptoms that may signal liver problems (e.g., unexplained fatigue, abdominal pain, loss of appetite, fever, vomiting, dark urine, pale stools, yellow eyes or skin). Not for use by persons under 18 years of age, or by pregnant or nursing women. Not for use with alcoholic beverages. Excessive use, or use with products that cause drowsiness, may impair your ability to operate a vehicle or dangerous equipment.

Mullein Garlic Ear Drops—for external use only; do not use in ears with perforated eardrums

Phytocillin®—if infection persists longer than three days or a fever is present, seek the advice of a primary care practitioner

Smoke Free®—large doses of the extract may cause nausea

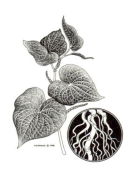

Kava

Deciding When to Avoid Certain Herbs 51

Vibrant Energy™—keep out of the reach of children

Q. Should I tell my doctor I am taking herbs?
Even though it might be difficult for you to talk to your doctor about the herbs that you are taking, I believe it is important to let him/her know. While some doctors may erroneously think that all herbs are dangerous or, conversely, have no effects, other physicians may be somewhat knowledgeable. Many are now learning about herbs. However, some are unsure where to find accurate and useful information, in which case sharing this book with your doctor may be helpful to both of you. Education is the key, and this book may provide them with a good source of information about herbal medicine.

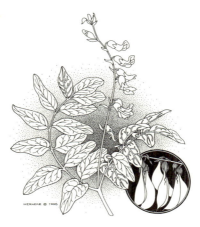

Astragalus

Chapter 6

Targeting Herbs for Specific Complaints

Q: What is the purpose of "targeting" herbal formulas?

"Targeting" aims at using the most therapeutically focused herbs for a precise health condition during a specific time frame. For more than 40 years, I have paid close attention to my clients, the herbs they were taking and the results they were getting. The recommendations in this chapter were born out of this experience as an herbalist. With the image of a dart game in mind, I visualize each herb as a dart and the condition to treat as a target. Bear in mind that as the disease progresses the target itself is constantly moving. Thus, an herb that may have been useful at the beginning of a disease may not offer much benefit once the disease is well established. Using an herbal formula that is specific for the stage of the illness and the condition of the tissue promotes the tissues back to health. Hitting the "bull's-eye" means you derive the maximum benefit from an herbal formula.

Q: Why should I target herbal formulas for specific health problems?

For example, Peak Defense™, an *Echinacea* and Goldenseal formula, used to treat colds and flu provides an example of how targeting gives you stronger, faster and longer-lasting results. Peak Defense™ is specific for subacute and chronic inflammation of mucous membranes. Thus, it is best used to combat the inflammation that starts around day two or three of a cold or flu. Use Peak Defense™ when mucous membrane inflammation has been present for a few days or more. Continue using it until all of your inflammatory symptoms are gone. Using Peak Defense™ in this way taps into 100 percent of its potential by hitting its bull's-eye.

However, in America, most products containing Goldenseal are used either for the prevention of colds and flu, or at the very beginning phases of these viral illnesses. Taking Goldenseal for these

Targeting Herbs for Specific Complaints

purposes is hitting the outer ring of the target, thus only 10 to 40 percent of Goldenseal's therapeutic benefits are being tapped, and the rest of the herb's benefits are wasted. There are many herbs that are far more appropriate for prevention of colds and flu and for the first day of a viral infection. For prevention consider herbs like medicinal mushrooms (Reishi, Shiitake, Maitake) found in Deep Health® while for the first few days of a cold or flu consider herbs like Andrographis, *Echinacea*, and Elder berry, found in Immune Alert™. Reserve Goldenseal, as found in Peak Defense™, for the mucous membrane inflammation that occurs on the second or third day of a cold or flu.

How to get the most out of this chapter:

Refer to the Herbal Directory (Chapter 7) for a description of what the formula is for, how it works, ingredients, suggested use, contraindications, possible side effects and warnings, when applicable, for each herbal formula. Pay special attention to the fact that several of the formulas recommended in these charts are contraindicated during pregnancy and some are contraindicated in nursing.

Herbs for Skin Problems

Skin problems can occur due to a multitude of factors including diet, stress, allergies, contact with irritating substances and monthly hormonal changes. Many of the drugs used for skin problems suppress symptoms so that the existing imbalance tends to recur shortly after the drugs are discontinued. In order to fully resolve skin problems, the way your body processes and eliminates waste products must be optimized.

In holistic herbal therapy, it is said that there is a ten to one ratio between the time an existing problem has been present and the time that it takes to heal the condition. For example, if you have had psoriasis for 20 years, it will take up to two years for your skin to become healthy and problem-free. Be aware that although it may take a few weeks to many months to change a habitual skin response, it will happen if patience and persistence are exercised.

Symptoms	Recommended Formulas
Bacterial infection (Strep, Staph, MRSA and others); bedsores; wounds; boils; infected cuts; impetigo	Phytocillin® (both internally and diluted externally)
Itching and insect bites of many kinds; jellyfish; Portuguese man-of-war	Bug Itch *ReLeaf*® (externally) Lymphatonic™ (internally)
Eczema; allergies	Allergy *ReLeaf*® System
Hives	Allertonic®
Fungus; lichen; athlete's foot; candida; diaper rash	Yeast *ReLeaf*® (internally and externally)
Herpes, labial or genital	Mouth Tonic™ (externally diluted)
Poison ivy; poison oak; contact dermatitis	Ivy Itch ReLeaf® (externally) Lymphatonic™ (internally)
Shingles, rash in	Phytocillin® (externally)
Shingles, pain in	Nervine Tonic™ (internally)

Herbs for Colds and Flu

In this table, the symptoms associated with colds and flu are listed in chronological order in terms of what unfolds in the body during this type of illness. To avoid a cold or the flu in the first place, use one of the two prevention formulas recommended. However, if you are getting or already have a cold or the flu, this table helps you choose the formula you need for your specific symptoms, at the point where you are in the viral or bacterial cycle. For instance, Peak Defense™ is great for combating inflammation on the second or third day of a cold or the flu. It is not as effective in stopping a cold or the flu in its first day (as Immune Alert™ is), or to cleanse the body after the illness is over (as Lymphatonic™ is).

Targeting Herbs for Specific Complaints 55

Symptoms	Recommended Formulas
Prevention; ongoing, year-round	Deep Health®
Prevention; one to two months before cold season and/or during stressful periods (traveling, long work hours, etc.)	ImmunoBoost™
Day one of cold/flu; malaise; aches, fever	Immune Alert™
Day two or three; cold; body aches, feeling rotten; sore throat & inflammation; stuffy sinuses	Peak Defense™
Day two or three; flu attacking lungs; flu-related pneumonia; acute viral bronchitis	Loviral™
Day four, five or six; acute lung conditions; cold/flu that's migrated to the lungs; thick mucus; cough	Respiratonic®
Day four, five or six; infection usually present, and mucus yellow or green	Phytocillin®
Day four, five or six; sore throat with laryngitis & pharyngitis	Singer's Saving Grace®
Day four, five or six; cold settled in head: dry membranes, stuffy nose, thick mucus	Congest Free™
Hard-to-shake or recurrent colds/flu; frequent colds or minor illnesses	Lymphatonic™

Herbs for Smoking Cessation

The first thing to consider when you want to stop smoking is your motivation. In my clinical experience, no amount of herbs will make up for weak motivation, especially when smokers try to quit in order to please others. If you truly want to quit for yourself out of choice, not obligation, then your likelihood of success dramatically increases. Because nicotine addiction affects the physiology of the body in several ways, it is best to provide yourself with herbal support in a variety of areas. This table lists symptoms in six challenged areas for individuals quitting smoking. The good news is that, unlike tobacco or nicotine drug products, none of these herbs is habit forming.

Symptoms	Recommended Formulas
Cravings, can't stand it another minute; need relief now	Smoke Free® Spray
Cravings, to reduce them throughout the day	Smoke Free® Softgels
Lung congestion; choking feeling with thick lung mucus	Respiratonic®
Nervous irritability; feeling as if you want to jump out of your skin; chattering or busy brain; insomnia	Stress *ReLeaf*®
Stressed endocrine system associated with cravings and low energy	Adrenotonic™

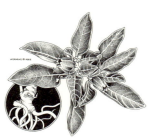

Ashwagandha

Targeting Herbs for Specific Complaints 57

Herbs for Allergies

Allergies, or allergic rhinitis, can be related to a multitude of seasonal and nonseasonal irritants ranging from tree pollens to house dust, as well as environmental and dietary factors. Thus, this is a difficult area to address from just one vantage point. Generally, in addition to herbal support, I urge you to take corrective measures to reduce stress in your life, since sinuses and nasal membranes react to overall health and stress levels. Improve your diet by favoring green and orange vegetables as well as brightly colored fruits. Avoid dairy products, gluten-containing grains (especially wheat), sugar, alcohol and sweets, which aggravate allergies, among other things. For additional suggestions on how to heal allergies naturally, I recommend my book *Breathe Free*, co-written with Amadea Morningstar and published by Lotus Press.

Stinging Nettle

Symptoms	Recommended Formulas
Hay fever; allergies to trees, flowers and ragweeds	Allergy *ReLeaf*® System
Prevention & support; adrenal gland support	Adrenotonic™
Liver support to process inflammatory waste products from allergic reaction	Liver Tonic™
Hay fever symptoms; thick mucus; congestion; no drainage	Congest Free™

Herbs for Digestive Problems

Optimal functioning of your digestion is intimately connected to what you eat. As stated in Chapter 1, *The Ten Elements of Great Health*, it is important for you to attend to the quality of your diet on a daily basis. Take a few minutes to relax before eating; relaxing encourages the flow of digestive juices to your gastrointestinal tract. If you are experiencing digestive distress, there are effective herbal formulas to improve digestive system function. Practice good dietary habits and support your herbal regimen by drinking plenty of water each day (one ounce for every two pounds of body weight up to a maximum of 64 ounces a day). Avoid iced drink with meals because it inhibits stomach function.

Symptoms	Recommended Formulas
Canker sores (aphthous stomatitis); pyorrhea	Mouth Tonic™
Stomach gas; bloating & burning sensation; colic; heartburn; indigestion	Stomach Tonic™
Stomach or intestinal cramping with possible diarrhea	Cramp *ReLeaf*®
Poor fat absorption; oily stools; dry skin; mild constipation	Liver Tonic™
Diarrhea; dysentery; entamoeba; giardia; pinworms	ParaFree™
Candida symptoms; thrush; dermatitis; diarrhea, flatulence & "sick all over" feeling	Yeast *ReLeaf*®
Digestive problems due to stress	Nervine Tonic™

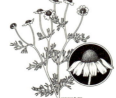

Chamomile

Targeting Herbs for Specific Complaints 59

Herbs for Women's Reproductive System

Women have always been a major force in support of herbal medicine. This support is due, in large part, to the fact that herbs offer a more harmonious and gentler way of working with the body than drugs. Herbs answer women's need to find safer, less intrusive and less disruptive treatments for female reproductive system issues.

Symptoms	Recommended Formulas
Menstrual cramps, sharp, stabbing pain	Cramp *ReLeaf*®
Menstrual cramps, dull; pain in muscles	Herbaprofen®
Breast, ovarian, and uterine cysts	Lymphatonic™
Menopausal symptoms	Menopautonic™
Urinary tract infection especially after sexual relations	CranBladder *ReLeaf*®
Frequent herpes outbreaks	Stress *ReLeaf*®
Candida; vaginitis; yeast infections	Yeast *ReLeaf*®

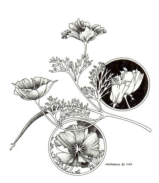

California Poppy

Herbs for Respiratory Problems

Many respiratory problems arise as an aftermath of colds and flu. Other imbalances may stem from long-term irritation of the pulmonary tissues by tobacco smoke, industrial dusts, and air pollution. This section's goal aims at keeping your respiratory system healthy all year round. The key to successfully beating lung problems is through the use of herbal support that addresses the specific needs of the respiratory system.

Symptoms	Recommended Formulas
Colds; chest congestion; chest cold; acute bronchitis; pleurisy	Respiratonic®
Flu; pneumonia; viral pulmonary infection; acute viral bronchitis	Loviral™
Bacterial respiratory infections; middle-ear, sinus, throat, or lung infections	Phytocillin®
Chronic bronchitis; emphysema; long-term management of ongoing lung problems	Lung Tonic™
Low red-blood-cell count; fatigue; low oxygen-blood saturation; shortness of breath; difficulty acclimating to high altitudes	ChlorOxygen®
Lung congestion; thick mucus; inflammation of throat, lungs & bronchioles; cough preventing sleep	Osha Root Throat Syrup
Day four, five, or six of a cold/flu; sore throat with laryngitis & pharyngitis	Singer's Saving Grace®
Seasonal, environmental, and dietary allergies affecting the lungs	Allergy *ReLeaf*® System
Smoking cessation support	Smoke Free®
Prevent or stop middle ear infection	Mullein Garlic Ear Drops

Chapter 7

Herbal Directory

Notes on this Herbal Directory:

This chapter lists herbal formulas and single herbs in alphabetic order. To find the herbal products that are best suited for your health issues, you can start by consulting the **Health Condition Index** (Chapter 9) which recommends the best herbal extracts for conditions ranging from Abdominal pain to Yeast infection, and then refer back to this chapter to look up the specific herbal formulas or single herbs you need.

Note that when an herb is designated as a "fresh herb" it means that the herb has not been dried prior to extraction. Also, for all formulas, ingredients are always listed in descending order of content. Please follow all suggested use recommendations, and pay attention to contraindications, possible side effects and/or warnings when applicable.

Adrenotonic™
What it's for: Use after corticosteroid therapy to strengthen adrenal gland function. Ideal for any illnesses that are aggravated during stressful periods, such as asthma, chronic fatigue immunodysfunction syndrome (CFIDS), hypoglycemia or allergies of all kinds. Supportive when facing increasing levels of responsibilities, lack of sleep, stressful situations or health challenges.
How it works: Superb adrenal gland tonic. Excellent adaptogen that increases resistance to a broad spectrum of physical, chemical or biological stressors.
Ingredients: Fresh Black Currant leaf, Astragalus root, Licorice root, Siberian Eleuthero root, cultivated American Ginseng root, Schisandra berry, Sarsaparilla root and Fo-ti cured root.
Suggested Use: Take one softgel or 25 drops with water twice a day. For maximum support take for at least 100 days or longer. May be taken indefinitely.
Contraindications: Do not use during pregnancy.

Allergy *ReLeaf*® System

What it's for: Seasonal hay fever, allergic rhinitis, itchy eyes, sneezing, inflammation of the mouth, stomach and/or intestines caused by allergies. Excellent in cases of allergies that manifest as eczema, hives, asthma, skin rash, sinusitis, headaches and diarrhea.

How it works: Stabilizes mast cells and calms their responses to airborne pollens and food allergens. Delivers essential nutrients and ongoing soothing comfort. Promotes a healthy allergenic response of the respiratory and digestive systems. Soothes temporary respiratory, digestive and skin irritation from environmental, dietary and seasonal challenges. maintains healthy eye, sinus, throat, lung, adrenal, skin and gastrointestinal tissues.

Ingredients: Each Allergy *ReLeaf*® System consists of two formulas—Allertonic® and Quercetin *AllerReLeaf*®. Allertonic® contains: fresh Stinging Nettle herb, Licorice root, Eyebright herb, Horehound herb, Osha root, fresh Horsetail herb, fresh Mullein leaf, Elecampane root and fresh Plantain leaf. Quercetin *AllerReLeaf*® contains: 500 mg Quercetin, 200 mg Vitamin C, 100 mg Pantothenic acid (Vitamin B5), 50 mg Turmeric (95% curcuminoids) and 50 mg Bromelain (2,400 GDU).

Suggested Use: **Acute:** Take one Allertonic® softgel and one Quercetin *AllerReLeaf*® tablet with water every two to three hours until comfort is achieved or as directed by your healthcare professional. Noticeable comfort is attained within the first or second day. Then switch to Ongoing use. **Ongoing:** Take one Allertonic® softgel and one Quercetin *AllerReLeaf*® tablet with water three times a day. **Proactive:** Two months prior to seasonal challenges, take one Allertonic® softgel and one Quercetin *AllerReLeaf*® tablet with water twice a day. **Best results are achieved when these two products are taken together.**

Allertonic®

What it's for: For allergies that manifest as eczema, hay fever, hives, asthma, skin rash, sinusitis, headaches, diarrhea, allergic rhinitis, chronic bronchitis, itchy eyes, sneezing, and inflammation of the mouth, stomach and/or intestines.

How it works: Supports healthy inflammatory responses of the respiratory and gastro-intestinal tracts. Stabilizes mast cell walls and fixed antibodies found in the eyes and respiratory system, keeping the tissues calm. Supports a healthy respiratory system by normalizing secretions, liquefying mucus, stimulating its removal from the lungs and keeping the pulmonary tissues hydrated.

Ingredients: Fresh Stinging Nettle herb, Licorice root, Eyebright herb, Horehound herb, Osha root, fresh Horsetail herb, fresh Mullein leaf, Elecampane root and fresh Plantain leaf.

Suggested Use: **Acute:** Take one softgel or 40 drops with water every two to three hours until comfort is achieved or as directed by your health care professional. Noticeable comfort is attained within the first or second day. Then switch to Ongoing use. **Ongoing:** Take one softgel or 40 drops with water three times a day. **Proactive:** Two months prior to seasonal challenges, take one softgel or 40 drops with water twice a day.

Bug Itch *ReLeaf*®
FOR EXTERNAL USE ONLY

What it's for: Provides relief from mosquito, noseum, spider, bee, wasp, insect stings, and bites. Also for sea creatures such as jellyfish and Portuguese man-of-war. Unlike creams or salves, no rubbing required, just spray.

How it works: Reduces inflammation of epidermis (skin). Offers specific protection against bacterial skin intruders. Strengthens skin resistance to enzymatic (such as hyaluronidase) damage caused by insect bites.

Ingredients: Echinacea angustifolia root, fresh Calendula flower, Propolis gum, fresh Plantain leaf and Licorice root.

Suggested Use: **FOR EXTERNAL USE ONLY.** Spray liberally on affected area(s) from three times a day up to every two hours, depending on severity of bites. To enhance results, take 30 drops or one softgel of Immune Alert™ with water three times a day or up to every two hours, depending on severity of bites or skin reaction.

ChlorOxygen® Chlorophyll Concentrate
(Extracted from Stinging Nettle)

What it's for: Use for low red blood cell count, fatigue, shortness of breath, high altitude sickness, or heavy menstrual flow. Useful during pregnancy when low hematocrit levels are present. Supportive for individuals with colostomies or intestinal gas.

How it works: Builds red blood cells. Increases hemoglobin's capacity to grab and distribute oxygen throughout the body. Helpful in high altitude situations. Supports pregnancy by maintaining healthy hematocrit levels. Acts as an intestinal deodorizer and offers liver protection.

Suggested Use: Take a daily total of 100-200 mg of ChlorOxygen® with water. Each 18 drops of liquid concentrate, and each softgel, delivers 50 mg of chlorophyll.

Flavors: Liquid concentrate also in mint flavor.

Side Effects: Dark green stools may occur.

Caution: Permanently stains fabric, building materials.

Congest Free™

What it's for: For sinus congestion with hot, dry membranes, headache, pain, pressure and heaviness in the sinuses, blocked ears, earache and bleeding nose from dryness. Opens up congested sinuses. Specific for thick mucus, difficulty blowing your nose and when it feels like your head is in a vise-like grip.

How it works: Supports sinus health. Balances sinus pressure. Good to use when traveling by plane while congested.

Ingredients: Xanthium fruit, Cassia twig, Magnolia bud, fresh Grindelia flower, Chinese Mint herb, Cubeb berry, Eyebright herb, Chinese Lovage root, Osha root and Cayenne fruit.

Suggested Use: Take 30 drops in water up to four times a day.

Contraindications: Do not use during pregnancy or while nursing.

Herbal Directory

Cramp *ReLeaf*® (menstrual)
What it's for: Relieves sharp, strong uterine or ovarian cramps occurring prior to or during menstruation. Eases uterine, ovarian and lower-abdominal muscle tension. For diarrhea and upset stomach that accompany menstruation.

How it works: Supports a healthy, normal monthly menstrual cycle. Improves ovarian and uterine circulation, soothes the pelvic muscles and promotes healthy tone of the entire birthing organ.

Ingredients: Black Haw stem bark, Cramp Bark bark, Bethroot root, Clove flower bud, Cinnamon bark, fresh Wild Yam root, Cardamom seed and Orange peel.

Suggested Use: Take one softgel or 40 drops (½ teaspoon) with water every three to four hours. Increase suggested use to 2 softgels or 80 drops (one teaspoon) with water per serving should you need or desire more support/relief.

Proactive: As a preventive measure take one softgel or 40 drops with water twice a day for five days prior to menstruation.

CranBladder *ReLeaf*®
What it's for: Prevents and stops recurring urinary tract infection (UTI), especially in females.

How it works: Maintains a healthy urinary tract and supports healthy bladder walls especially when the urine is strongly acidic or alkaline. Supports the secretion of bacterial anti-adherence factors. Keeps the mucous lining of the urinary system healthy. Stimulates the urinary tract immune system and tones the urinary passages.

Ingredients: Cranberry fruit, Uva-ursi leaf, *Echinacea angustifolia* root, fresh Stinging Nettle herb, Buchu leaf, fresh Horsetail herb, Pipsissewa herb, fresh Yarrow flowering top, Meadowsweet herb, Licorice root and Stevia herb.

Suggested Use: **Acute**: Take 1 softgel or 30 drops with water every two to three hours. **Ongoing**: Take 1 softgel or 30 drops with water twice a day.

Contraindications: Do not use during pregnancy.

Side Effects: Peculiar urine smell and color may occur.

Deep Health®

What it's for: A daily multi-herbal and long-term preventive formula. Offers ongoing support during long standing, serious or debilitating health challenges. Helps relieve nervousness, anxiety, sleeplessness. Offers support in chronic hepatitis, allergies, stomach and intestinal ulcers, as well as chronic respiratory problems such as asthma, emphysema and bronchitis. Useful to reduce high cholesterol and high triglyceride levels. Stabilizes blood sugar problems. Use in lack of sleep, decreased resistance due to hectic lifestyle, frequent travels, jet lag, demanding work or social schedule.

How it works: Excellent deep immune system tonic. Possesses substantial adaptogenic and immune modulating properties. Supports the health of internal organs including heart, liver, stomach, intestines, lungs, pancreas, kidneys, and adrenal glands, as well as circulatory and nervous systems. Improves endurance and physical performance, protects against stress, decreases fatigue, and promotes calmness, energy and vitality.

Ingredients: Reishi mushroom fruiting body, Shiitake mushroom fruiting body, California Spikenard root, Astragalus root, Maitake mushroom fruiting body, Ashwagandha root, Siberian Eleuthero root, Schisandra berry, Cordyceps mushroom mycelium and Ginger root.

Suggested Use: As a daily multi-herbal dietary supplement take one softgel or 40 drops with water twice a day, every day.

Deep Sleep®

What it's for: Specific for inability to fall asleep, waking up frequently during the night with difficulty returning to sleep, waking up too early in the morning or experiencing unrefreshing sleep. For insomnia resulting from depression, for waking up groggy or tired, as well as for fitful and/or agitated sleep. For sleep problems accompanied by cramps or pain. For insomnia occuring while weaning from drugs, alcohol or cigarettes. Also for inability to fall asleep from excessive tiredness.

How it works: Reduces sleep latency (amount of time required to fall asleep) and stops excessive

mind chatter. Reeducates the brain's sleep center and creates positive sleep patterns. It is not habit forming, has no side effects and does not interfere with REM (rapid eye movement) sleep.
Ingredients: Fresh California Poppy plant, fresh Valerian root, fresh Passionflower herb tip, fresh Chamomile flower, fresh Lemon Balm herb, fresh Oat seed in milky stage and Orange peel.
Suggested Use: Take one softgel or 30 drops with a little water one hour before bedtime and again at bedtime. Best results are achieved by the second or third night.

Deprezac™
What it's for: Specific for mild to moderate depression. For mild anxiety, tension, fatigue, irritability, sleep problems, agitation, loss of appetite, loss of interest and excessive sleeping. Supportive for seasonal affective disorder (SAD).
How it works: Helps maintain a positive mental outlook. Possesses relaxing, calming and uplifting properties.
Ingredients: St. John's Wort herb in bud stage, fresh Lemon Balm herb, Schisandra berry, fresh Oat seed in milky stage, fresh Peppermint herb, fresh Valerian root, Siberian Eleuthero root, fresh Rosemary leaf, Damiana leaf and Stevia herb.
Suggested Use: Take 30 drops in water three times a day for three weeks then 30 drops twice a day in water for at least six months.
Contraindication: Do not use during pregnancy or while nursing. Do not use with HIV protease inhibitors, cyclosporine, warfarin, digoxin and many other drugs.
Warning: Do not use in bipolar syndrome and/or for any other severe depressive states. Consult with your primary care physician if you are taking other medications.

Early Alert™ see Immune Alert™

Echinacea Triple Source™
What it's for: A complete spectrum full-potency formula. A first response immune system activator. Ideal for the initial stages of colds and flu.
How it works: Stimulates production, matura-

tion, mobilization and aggressiveness of white blood cells and other body defenses against possible viruses or bacteria. Strengthens the connective tissues and maintains healthy tendons, joints and articulations. Strengthens throat tissues and increases its resistance when faced with seasonal challenges.

Ingredients: Dried *Echinacea angustifolia* and *pallida* root, fresh *Echinacea angustifolia* and *purpurea* root, fresh *Echinacea angustifolia* and *purpurea* herb and flower, and *Echinacea purpurea* seed.

Suggested Use: **Acute:** At the first sign of cold or flu take 40 drops with water every hour. Ongoing: Take 30 drops with water twice a day.

Essiac Tonic

Originally given to Canadian nurse René Caisse by an Ojibwa (Chippewa) Indian to eradicate cancer.

What it's for: Alleviates chronic and degenerative diseases. Offers ongoing support in autoimmune disorders, allergic disorders, and chronic fatigue immuno-dysfunction syndrome (CFIDS).

How it works: Supportive formula during physically stressful times. Moves the body toward a state of integration and health. Eliminates waste products and restores challenged cells to health. Boosts the immune system. Cleanses and supports the liver and blood.

Ingredients: Burdock root, Sheep Sorrel herb, Slippery Elm inner bark and Chinese (Turkey) Rhubarb root.

Suggested Use: Take one softgel or 30 drops with water twice a day on an empty stomach.

Contraindications: Do not use during pregnancy.

HB Pressure™ Tonic

What it's for: Helpful in cases of mild to moderately elevated blood pressure. Especially helpful when high blood pressure is due to stress or is aggravated by excessive sodium intake. Useful in either systolic or diastolic elevations.

How it works: Supports healthy blood pressure. Promotes healthy systolic and diastolic pressure. Dilates blood vessels, including coronary blood vessels. Reduces peripheral resistance. Enhances healthy cholesterol metabolism.

Herbal Directory 69

Ingredients: Linden flower, European Mistletoe leaf twig, fresh Dandelion leaf, fresh Passionflower herb tip, Hawthorn berry, Siberian Eleuthero root, fresh Yarrow flower top, fresh Skullcap herb, Prickly Ash bark and Hawthorn leaf and flower.
Suggested Use: Take one softgel or 30 drops with water three times a day.
Contraindications: Do not use during pregnancy.
Side Effects: May cause low blood pressure.
Warning: Monitor your blood pressure to ensure that this herbal approach is effective for you.

Herbaprofen®
What it's for: Reduces pain and spasms caused by toothaches, uterine and fallopian tube cramps, neuralgia, intestinal colic, gallstones and renal colics, rheumatoid arthritis, fibrositis, sore muscles, spasmodic cough, sciatica, sprained back, etc. Useful for congestive headaches. Beneficial when pain prevents sleep.
How it works: An excellent support for muscular health. Balances harmful and beneficial inflammatory compounds. Reduces excessive tension of voluntary and involuntary muscles. Eases spasms of skeletal and smooth muscles. Promotes relaxation.
Ingredients: Jamaica Dogwood bark, Black Cohosh root, fresh Betony herb, Meadowsweet herb, fresh Passionflower herb tip, Devil's Claw root, Licorice root and Stevia herb.
Suggested Use: Take 40 drops with water up to every three hours or as needed.
Contraindications: Do not use during pregnancy or while nursing.

Immune Alert™
(formerly Early Alert™)
What it's for: Ideal for the initial stages of seasonal immune system challenges, colds and at the beginning of a general infection. Prevents or slows down bacterial and viral infections. Boosts the immune system prior to cold and flu season. Reduces swelling and stimulates repair in tendonitis, bursitis, tennis elbow and other sports injuries. Also for tonsillitis, herpes, respiratory system infection, candida, thrush and contact dermatitis.

How it works: A first-response immune system activator. Stimulates the production, maturation, mobilization and aggressiveness of white blood cells and other body defenses against possible intruders. Strengthens connective tissues and maintains healthy tendons, joints and articulations. Strengthens throat tissues and increases their resistance against the infiltration of microorganisms.

Ingredients: Andrographis herb, dried *Echinacea angustifolia* and *pallida* roots, fresh *Echinacea angustifolia* and *purpurea* root, fresh *Echinacea angustifolia* and *purpurea* herb and flower, dried *Echinacea purpurea* mature seeds, Olive leaf, fresh Elder berry and fresh Spilanthes herb.

Suggested Use: **Acute:** At the very first sign of a seasonal challenge take one softgel or 30 drops with water every hour. **Ongoing:** Take one softgel or 30 drops with water twice a day.

ImmunoBoost™

What it's for: Use during the change of seasons to support and boost the immune system. Prevents colds and flu. Builds the immune system during stressful times or while traveling. Prevents recurring middle ear infections (otitis media) in children. Also for acute tonsillitis, genital or oral herpes, upper respiratory tract infection. For chronic yeast infection, thrush and contact dermatitis.

How it works: Builds a fast-acting and proactive immune system. Boosts immune system by increasing interferon production which alerts the body at the first sign of a challenge. Prepares the body to deal with future intruders. Reduces occurrence of middle-ear infections in children.

Ingredients: Dried *Echinacea angustifolia* root, fresh *Echinacea angustifolia* root, herb and flower, fresh *Echinacea purpurea* root, Astragalus root, Osha root, *Echinacea purpurea* seed and fresh Calendula flower.

Suggested Use: As a preventive take one softgel or 30 drops with water twice a day for at least one month. For chronic or recurring conditions take one softgel or 30 drops with water three times a day until condition resolves.

Ivy Itch ReLeaf®
FOR EXTERNAL USE ONLY

What it's for: Soothes plant caused skin irritations in sensitive individuals. Useful for poison ivy, poison oak, poison sumac, stinging nettle, mullein and other plant skin irritations. Used for herpes outbreaks (mouth or genital).

How it works: Soothes affected skin areas. Decreases inflammation of the skin surfaces. Relieves intense itching. Stimulates skin healing of challenged areas. Unlike creams or salves, no rubbing required—just spray.

Ingredients: Fresh Jewel weed herb, fresh Grindelia flower, fresh Plantain leaf, Licorice root and *Echinacea angustifolia* root.

Suggested Use: Spray liberally on affected areas from three times a day or up to every two hours in acute situations. Let dry.

Warning: **FOR EXTERNAL USE ONLY.** Discontinue use and consult with a doctor if condition persists, worsens or an infection occurs.

Kava Cool Complex™

What it's for: Promotes emotional well-being. Useful for mild to moderate anxiety, edginess, tension, mental and physical agitation. Relieves nervousness and tension due to stress. Permits sleep when insomnia is due to muscle tightness, mental tension or agitation.

How it works: Supports a positive mental outlook. Possesses mood-elevating properties, anxiolytic actions and counters anxiety by relaxing mind and body. Decreases a person's perceived level of stress without interfering with clear, focused thinking.

Ingredients: Kava root, Chamomile flower, St. John's Wort herb in bud, fresh Oat seed in the milky stage, fresh Passionflower herb tip, Hops strobile, fresh Skullcap herb and Stevia herb.

Suggested Use: Take one softgel or 30 drops with water as needed.

Contraindications: Do not use during pregnancy or while nursing. Do not use with alcohol or barbiturates.

Side Effects: Very large amounts over an extended period of time may cause skin rash.

Warning: US FDA advises that a potential risk of rare, but severe, liver injury may be associated with kava-containing dietary supplements. Ask a healthcare professional before use if you have or have had liver problems, frequently use alcoholic beverages, or are taking any medication. Stop use and see a doctor if you develop symptoms that may signal liver problems (e.g., unexplained fatigue, abdominal pain, loss of appetite, fever, vomiting, dark urine, pale stools, yellow eyes or skin). Not for use by persons under 18 years of age, or by pregnant or nursing women. Not for use with alcoholic beverages. Excessive use, or use with products that cause drowsiness, may impair your ability to operate a vehicle or dangerous equipment.

Note: If taken for depression, consider alternating with Deprezac™.

Kidney Tonic™

What it's for: For nonspecific inflammation of the kidneys or bladder, lower back pain, water retention in PMS or from changes in heat or humidity. Use in bacterial infection of the urethra or bladder and irritation of the urethra after sex. Useful for frequent, urgent, burning or painful urination. Helpful for pain in the pubic area and the tendency to urinate excessively at night.

How it works: Promotes healthy kidney and bladder function, and when used over a long period of time, strengthens the urinary system.

Ingredients: Fresh Dandelion leaf, fresh Saw Palmetto berry, Parsley root, Couch Grass root, Boldo leaf, Buchu leaf, Juniper berry, Uva-ursi leaf, Pipsissewa herb and Cubeb berry.

Suggested Use: **Acute:** Take one softgel or 30 drops with water every four hours. **Ongoing:** Take one softgel or 20 drops with water twice a day.

Contraindications: Do not use during pregnancy.

Notice: Peculiar urine smell and color may occur.

Liver Tonic™

What it's for: Use when there are elevated liver enzymes (SGOT, SGPT), difficulty digesting fats, or during hepatitis flare-ups. Useful for mild frontal headaches after fatty meals, alcohol, coffee or chocolate; mild constipation and simple jaundice. Suggested for individuals who have been or are exposed to aromatic hydrocarbons

such as solvents, paints, thinners, etc.
How it works: Activates Kupffer's cells in the liver to for break down and eliminate waste products. Lowers high bilirubin levels. Protects liver cells against toxins. Stimulates repair of liver cells. Supports liver and gallbladder health.
Ingredients: Milk Thistle seed, fresh Toadflax herb, Oregon Grape root, *Echinacea angustifolia* root, Licorice root, fresh Celandine herb, Fringe Tree root bark, Culver's Root root and Blue Flag root.
Suggested Use: Take one softgel or 20 drops with water three times a day.
Contraindications: Do not use during pregnancy.

Loviral™
What it's for: Specific to prevent pneumonia or other lung infections that often occur in the second stage of a cold or flu. Useful for fevers that accompany colds or flu, congested lungs, acute bronchitis, tonsillopharyngitis, sore throat, thick mucus, dry cough and irritated cough.
How it works: Supports healthy sinuses, throat, lungs and pulmonary tissues during colds and flu season. Enhances function of immune and respiratory systems. Thins and loosens mucus, promotes expectoration and ensures strong immune response against viral and bacterial respiratory microorganisms.
Ingredients: Lomatium root, Pelargonium root, Osha root, fresh Elder berry, Andrographis herb, Honeysuckle flower, fresh Grindelia flower, Elecampane root, *Echinacea angustifolia* root, Licorice root, fresh Elder flower, fresh Yarrow flower top, fresh Lobelia herb in bladder seed stage.
Suggested Use: Take one softgel or 30 drops with water every two to three hours until lung health is restored.
Contraindications: Do not use during pregnancy.
Side Effects: May cause a skin rash.
Discontinue use if rash occurs.

Lung Tonic™
What it's for: Ideal formula for long-term management of lung problems. Support for chronic obstructive pulmonary disease (COPD), including emphysema, chronic bronchitis and asthma.

Useful for congestion, inflammation of bronchioles and lung tissue, spasms of bronchioles and excessive production of mucus. Prevents respiratory infection, soothes and calms coughs.

How it works: Specific for long-term use. Supports healthy lung function. Promotes long-term respiratory support in chronic and prolonged lung challenges. Maximizes lung capacity. Enhances oxygen absorption. Strengthens and opens up the respiratory passages.

Ingredients: Fresh Mullein leaf, Horehound herb, Elecampane root, fresh Grindelia flower, *Echinacea angustifolia* root, Pleurisy Root root, fresh Passionflower herb tip, Osha root, fresh Lobelia herb in bladder seed stage and Yerba Santa leaf.

Suggested Use: Take one softgel or 30 drops with water three times a day.

Lymphatonic™

What it's for: A must for recurring or lingering, hard-to-shake infections, colds, flu, and frequent minor illnesses. Use for acute swelling of tonsils and/or lymph nodes. Specific for uterine, ovarian or breast cysts. Speeds up healing of cuts, boils, herpes, shingles or other poorly healing abrasions. Shortens healing time of poison ivy or poison oak infection as well as cat-scratch disease.

How it works: Promotes healthy lymphatic function. Deep-acting immune system cleanser. Stimulates fluid drainage from congested tissues including drainage of uterine, ovarian or breast tissues. Supports healing of skin abrasions and infections.

Ingredients: *Echinacea angustifolia* root, Red Root root, Ocotillo stem bark, Burdock root, Licorice root, fresh Dandelion root, Yellow Dock root, Wild Indigo root, Blue Flag root and Stillingia root.

Suggested Use: Take one softgel or 30 drops with water three times a day.

Contraindications: Do not use during pregnancy.

Menopautonic™

What it's for: Decreases or stops menopausal symptoms such as hot flashes, night sweats, nervousness, insomnia, urinary frequency,

Herbal Directory 75

vaginal dryness and back pain. Lifts menopausal depression.
How it works: Eases menopausal transition and enhances post menopausal health. Normalizes female hormonal system. Strengthens the heart and nervous system.
Ingredients: Dong Quai cured root, Vitex berry, fresh Hawthorn leaf and flower, fresh Motherwort herb, Licorice root, fresh Passionflower herb tip, Black Cohosh root, Siberian Eleuthero root, Pipsissewa herb and cultivated American Ginseng root.
Suggested Use: Take one softgel or 30 drops with water early morning and before retiring.
Contraindications: Do not use during pregnancy.

Migra-Free®
What it's for: Effective in migraine headache attacks, including those resistant to conventional medicines. Used daily, acts as a preventative.
How it works: Normalizes fatty acid metabolism ensuring healthy inflammatory response of brain, head and joint tissues. Enhances blood vessel stability. Taken every day, it stabilizes blood vessels and promotes healthy brain/blood circulation, thus acting as a preventive formula.
Ingredients: Fresh Feverfew herb, fresh Lesser Periwinkle herb, fresh Ginkgo leaf, Meadowsweet herb, White Willow bark and Stevia herb.
Suggested Use: **Acute:** Take 40 drops in water every hour. As a preventive take 40 drops in water once a day. Can be taken on an ongoing basis.

Mouth Tonic™
What it's for: Use as an external treatment for mouth and gum sores, bleeding gums, fever blisters, herpes sores, mouth ulcers (aphthous stomatitis), sores from dentures, enlarged and spongy tonsils and receding gums due to tissue degeneration. Also for pyorrhea and periodontal disease.
How it works: Promotes gum and oral tissue health. Stimulates circulation and regeneration of mouth lining. Promotes healthy tissues with denture, braces, or bridge use.
Ingredients: Echinacea angustifolia root, Myrrh

gum resin, Goldenseal root, Propolis gum, Yerba Mansa root and Bloodroot root.

Suggested Use: Apply with cotton swab twice a day. Do not rinse. If stinging or irritation occurs, dilute with a little water. Also use with water pick, cotton swab or toothbrush to maintain or restore periodontal health.

Warning: Do not use if you are allergic to bees or bee products.

Mushroom Seven Source™

What it's for: The ultimate medicinal mushroom formula. Offers support prior to and after surgery, chemotherapy and radiation therapy. Stabilizes blood sugar. Helpful with nervousness, anxiety and sleeplessness.

How it works: Deep immune system tonic. Supports and strengthens internal organs including lung, heart, liver, kidneys, stomach, pancreas, spleen, bladder, reproductive organ function, intestines, and nervous system. Supports healthy blood pressure. Protects stomach, respiratory and intestinal linings. Normalizes inflammatory response.

Ingredients: Reishi fruiting body, Shiitake fruiting body, Maitake fruiting body, Oyster fruiting body, Agaricus fruiting body, Tremella fruiting body and Cordyceps mycelium (may contain soy).

Suggested Use: Take 30 drops in water twice a day. For maximum support take for at least 100 days or longer. May be taken indefinitely.

Nervine Tonic™

What it's for: Useful for soothing muscle twitches, nervousness, anxiety, nervous tics, muscle tightness from stress or overexertion, muscle pain and intestinal cramps.

How it works: An all-purpose daily sedative. Soothes irritability of the nervous system and stimulates its repair.

Ingredients: Fresh Passionflower herb tip, fresh Valerian root, fresh Oat seed in milky stage, Black Cohosh root, fresh Skullcap herb and fresh Betony herb.

Suggested Use: Take 30 drops in water every three to four hours.

Contraindications: Do not use during pregnancy.

Herbal Directory

Osha Root Throat Syrup
What it's for: Stops or calms cough. Useful in lung congestion, inflammation of throat and bronchioles as well as dry scratchy throat.
How it works: Soothes throat irritation. Provides a protective coating to the throat tissues. Dilates the bronchioles, activates the movement of the cilia, decreases lung congestion, liquefies lung secretions and promotes expectoration.
Ingredients: Osha root, White Pine bark, Black Cherry bark, Spikenard root, Balsam Poplar bud and Bloodroot root in an evaporated cane juice syrup base.
Suggested Use: Take 1 teaspoon to 1 tablespoon every three to four hours. Children, two to five years old, take 1/2 to 1 teaspoon every three to four hours.
Contraindications: Do not use during pregnancy.

ParaFree™
What it's for: Eliminates parasites such as giardia, entamoeba, protozoa, pinworms and other types of parasites.
How it works: Promotes healthy digestive function. Tones gastrointestinal system. Useful as a biannual intestinal cleanser. Recommended for individuals who travel to foreign countries or are exposed to questionable water and food sources.
Ingredients: Fresh Black Walnut "green" hull (tree-nut), Wormwood herb, Quassia inner wood, Clove flower bud and Male Fern root.
Suggested Use: Take one softgel or 40 drops with water three times a day before meals.
Contraindications: Do not use during pregnancy or while nursing.

Peak Defense™
Formerly Goldenseal/Echinacea Complex
What it's for: Specific for the 2nd or 3rd day and beyond of a cold or flu. Breaks fevers. Liquefies mucus, relieves deep-seated joint, muscle and bone pains, headaches, and generalized body aches.
How it works: Stimulates the immune system's response. Strengthens the mucous membranes of the throat, sinus and bronchioles. Opens up sweat pores, stimulates waste product elimination and returns body to normal temperature. Helps the body return to optimal health.

Ingredients: Goldenseal root, *Echinacea angustifolia* root, Licorice root, Yerba Mansa root, fresh Yarrow flower top, fresh Elder flower, fresh Elder berry, Bayberry root bark, fresh Dandelion root, fresh Grindelia flower, Ginger root, Red Root root and Osha root.

Suggested Use: Take 1 softgel or 30 drops with water three to five times a day.

Contraindications: Do not use during pregnancy.

Phytocillin®

What it's for: **Internally:** Specific for bacterial infections. Resolves lingering cold and flu conditions. Use for sinus, throat, lungs, bronchioles, mouth, gum, stomach or intestinal bacterial infections. Use internally for Gram-positive bacterial infections and fungal infections. **Externally:** For bacterial infections (staph or strep) or fungal infection, athlete's foot, ringworm or as a douche in trichomonas infection. Also for abrasions, skin ulcers, boils, pressure ulcers (i.e.: bedsores), impetigo, skin infections or burns.

How it works: Inhibits bacterial or fungal growth. Promotes protective skin responses to outside challenges. Stimulates skin (epithelial) regeneration.

Ingredients: Usnea lichen, Yerba Mansa root, Propolis gum, *Echinacea angustifolia* root, Licorice root, Oregon Grape root and Hops strobile.

Suggested Use: **Acute:** Take two softgels or 60 drops with water five times a day until the infection is no longer noticeable. Continue this dosage for an additional two days to ensure complete elimination of resistant bacteria. **Externally:** Dilute half and half with water and apply.

Contraindications: Do not use during pregnancy.

Warning: Do not use if you are allergic to bees or bee products. If challenge persists longer than three days or a fever is present, seek the advice of a primary care practitioner.

Prostatonic™

What it's for: Relieves benign enlargement of the prostate when enlargement has caused varying degrees of urinary problems such as frequent and urgent urination, difficulty in urinating or sensation of incomplete emptying of the bladder and drib-

bling. Reduces inflammation of these tissues and increases uptake of circulating male hormones.
How it works: Supports healthy prostate function. Contributes to normal urination. Balances harmful and beneficial inflammatory compound in these tissues (prostaglandins) and increases uptake of circulating male hormones.
Ingredients: Fresh Saw Palmetto berry, fresh Yarrow flower top, Dong Quai cured root, fresh Stinging Nettle root, Damiana leaf, cultivated American Ginseng root, fresh Cleavers herb, Pipsissewa herb, Yerba Mansa root and Sarsaparilla root.
Suggested Use: Take 20-30 drops with water two to three times a day for an unlimited period of time. May take up to six weeks for effects to become noticeable.

Respiratonic®
What it's for: Specific for acute lung conditions. Relieves chest colds, lung congestion, acute bronchitis and pleurisy. Decreases excessive heat in the lungs, eases coughs and liquefies mucus.
How it works: Promotes healthy respiratory function. An all-purpose expectorant that loosens mucus secretions and soothes the respiratory passages. It hydrates lung tissues, dilates bronchioles and stimulates general lung immune resistance.
Ingredients: Echinacea angustifolia root, Osha root, Licorice root, Yerba Mansa root, Yerba Santa leaf, Pleurisy Root root, fresh Grindelia flower and Ginger root.
Suggested Use: Take one softgel or 30 drops with water three to five times a day.
Contraindications: Do not use during pregnancy.

Singer's® Citrus & Honey (Non-Alcohol)
What it's for: Ideal for sore throats, laryngitis, pharyngitis, hoarseness, cough, expectoration of thick mucus and a feeling of dryness in the throat. A blessing for singers, preachers, teachers or anyone with a sore throat from singing, screaming, cheering, shouting or talking loudly for a long period of time.
How it works: Promotes voice clarity and vocal comfort. Moistens and lubricates throat tissues.

Soothes feeling of throat dryness.

Ingredients: Extracts of Yerba Mansa root, fresh Stoneroot root, Licorice root, Jack-in-the-pulpit root, *Echinacea angustifolia* root and Ginger root. Flavors: lemon and lime essential oils, and citral.

Suggested Use: Spray throat two times per application as needed. Do not exceed 20 applications per day.

Contraindications: Do not use during pregnancy.

Caution: Sample any new throat product at least one day before using your voice professionally.

Singer's® Cool Mint

What it's for: Ideal for sore throats, laryngitis, pharyngitis, hoarseness, cough, expectoration of thick mucus and a feeling of dryness in the throat. A blessing for singers, preachers, teachers or anyone with a sore throat from singing, screaming, cheering, shouting or talking loudly for a long period of time.

How it works: Promotes voice clarity and vocal comfort. Moistens and lubricates throat tissues. Soothes feeling of throat dryness.

Ingredients: Extracts of Yerba Mansa root, fresh Stoneroot root, Licorice root, Jack-in-the-pulpit root, Propolis gum, *Echinacea angustifolia* root, and Ginger root. Flavors: menthol, vanilla flavoring, essential oils of eucalyptus, lemon, peppermint, and spearmint.

Suggested Use: Spray throat two times per application as needed. Do not exceed 20 applications per day.

Contraindications: Do not use during pregnancy.

Caution: Do not use if you are allergic to bees or bee products. Sample any new throat product at least one day before using your voice professionally.

Singer's® Extra Strentgh

What it's for: Ideal for sore throats, laryngitis, pharyngitis, hoarseness, cough, expectoration of thick mucus and a feeling of dryness in the throat. A blessing for singers, preachers, teachers or anyone with a sore throat from singing, screaming, cheering, shouting or talking loudly for a long period of time. Also for sore throats at the beginning of a cold or as an aftermath of a lung infection.

How it works: Promotes voice clarity and vocal comfort. Moistens and lubricates throat tissues. Soothes feeling of throat dryness.
Ingredients: Extracts of Yerba Mansa root, fresh Stoneroot root, Licorice root, Osha root, Jack-in-the-pulpit root, Propolis gum, *Echinacea angustifolia* root, and Ginger root.
Suggested Use: Spray throat two times per application as needed. Do not exceed 20 applications per day.
Contraindications: Do not use during pregnancy.
Caution: Do not use if you are allergic to bees or bee products. Sample any new throat product at least one day before using your voice professionally.

Singer's® Honey Lemon
What it's for: Ideal for sore throats, laryngitis, pharyngitis, hoarseness, cough, expectoration of thick mucus and a feeling of dryness in the throat. A blessing for singers, preachers, teachers or anyone with a sore throat from singing, screaming, cheering, shouting or talking loudly for a long period of time.
How it works: Promotes voice clarity and vocal comfort. Moistens and lubricates throat tissues. Soothes feeling of throat dryness.
Ingredients: Extracts of Yerba Mansa root, fresh Stoneroot root, Licorice root, Jack-in-the-pulpit root, Propolis gum, *Echinacea angustifolia* root, and Ginger root. Flavors: lemon and lime essential oils, and citral.
Suggested Use: Spray throat two times per application as needed. Do not exceed 20 applications per day.
Contraindications: Do not use during pregnancy.
Caution: Do not use if you are allergic to bees or bee products. Sample any new throat product at least one day before using your voice professionally.

Singer's® Professional Strength (Non-Alcohol)
What it's for: Ideal for sore throats, laryngitis, pharyngitis, hoarseness, cough, expectoration of thick mucus and a feeling of dryness in the throat. A blessing for singers, preachers, teachers or anyone with a sore throat from singing, screaming,

cheering, shouting or talking loudly for a long period of time. Also for sore throats at the beginning of a cold or as an aftermath of a lung infection.
How it works: Promotes voice clarity and vocal comfort. Moistens and lubricates throat tissues. Soothes feeling of throat dryness.
Ingredients: Extracts of Yerba Mansa root, fresh Stoneroot root, Licorice root, Osha root, Jack-in-the-pulpit root, *Echinacea angustifolia* root and Ginger root.
Suggested Use: Spray throat two times per application as needed. Do not exceed 20 applications per day.
Contraindications: Do not use during pregnancy.
Caution: Sample any new throat product at least one day before using your voice professionally.

Singer's® Serious Cinnamon
What it's for: Ideal for sore throats, laryngitis, pharyngitis, hoarseness, cough, expectoration of thick mucus and a feeling of dryness in the throat. A blessing for singers, preachers, teachers or anyone with a sore throat from singing, screaming, cheering, shouting or talking loudly for a long period of time.
How it works: Promotes voice clarity and vocal comfort. Moistens and lubricates throat tissues. Soothes feeling of throat dryness.
Ingredients: Extracts of Yerba Mansa root, fresh Stoneroot root, Licorice root, Jack-in-the-pulpit root, Propolis gum, *Echinacea angustifolia* root, and Ginger root. Flavors: cinnamon essential oil, vanilla extract, and sweet orange essential oil.
Suggested Use: Spray throat two times per application as needed. Do not exceed 20 applications per day.
Contraindications: Do not use during pregnancy.
Caution: Do not use if you are allergic to bees or bee products. Sample any new throat product at least one day before using your voice professionally.

Smoke Free®
What it's for: Curbs nicotine cravings. Decreases nervousness, edginess, irritability, and inability to relax when giving up tobacco. Alleviates lung congestion.

Herbal Directory 83

How it works: Assists the determined person who wishes to stop smoking. Decreases withdrawal symptoms, calms the nervous system, dilates the bronchioles and loosens mucus. Not habit forming.

Ingredients: Fresh Lobelia herb in bladder stage, fresh Oat seed in milky stage, Osha root, Licorice root, fresh Passionflower herb tip, Pleurisy Root root, fresh Grindelia flower, fresh Mullein leaf and Ginger root.

Suggested Use: Take one softgel with water every two to three hours and/or spray two times in mouth when smoking urge arises.

Contraindications: Excessive use may cause nausea. Do not use during pregnancy or while nursing. Keep out of the reach of children.

Stomach Tonic™
What it's for: Offers immediate relief for bloating, gas cramps, pain after eating, stomach acidity. Soothes stomach discomfort and sweetens the breath. Dispels nausea and vomiting.

How it works: Calms gastric tissues between meals and during the night.

Ingredients: Chamomile flower, fresh Catnip flower top, Fennel seed, fresh Lavender flower, Star Anise seed, Cardamom seed, Gentian root, Angelica root and Prickly Ash bark.

Suggested Use: For adults, take 30 drops in water three times a day, after meals or before bedtime. For babies, give 4 drops, diluted in a liquid, up to three times a day, after meals or before bedtime.

Contraindications: Do not use during pregnancy.

Stress ReLeaf®
What it's for: Especially useful for individuals faced with, or recuperating from, increased amounts of stress or prolonged period of elevated stress. Use for nervousness, edginess, anxiety, restlessness, panic attacks, exhaustion, nervous stomach, gastrointestinal tension or cramps, stress-related insomnia, muscle twitches, muscle pain or tightness, stress-induced high blood pressure, and stress-induced asthma.

How it works: Dual-acting protective formula delivers immediate stress-relieving effects and long-term coping benefits. Possesses calming and adaptogenic properties. Strengthens the body's resistance to the debilitating effects of elevated adrenaline. Shields and tones the nervous system, reduces tension, decreases nervous system irritation, promotes relaxation, and supports healthy adrenal gland function against the negative effects of stress.

Ingredients: Holy Basil [Krishna and Rama tulsi] herb, fresh Passionflower herb tip, fresh Valerian root, fresh Oat seed in milky stage, Ashwagandha root, Black Cohosh root, fresh Skullcap herb and fresh Betony herb.

Suggested Use: Take one softgel or 40 drops with water three times a day.

Contraindications: Do not use during pregnancy.

Ultimate Ginseng™

What it's for: Excellent for emotional or physical exhaustion, as a tonic after a prolonged illness or in depression from neurological or autoimmune disease. Use to prepare for or recuperate from major stress. Use as a tonic/adaptogen during challenging times.

How it works: Enhances stamina. Excellent adaptogenic formula to support, enhance well being, and maintain emotional and physical balance.

Ingredients: Woodsgrown American Ginseng root, wild American Ginseng root, Asian Kirin red Ginseng root, Asian white Ginseng root, cultivated American Ginseng root, and Siberian Eleuthero root.

Suggested Use: Take one softgel or 30 drops with water twice a day for at least one month to achieve best results.

Contraindications: Do not use during pregnancy.

Vibrant Energy™

What it's for: Helps you stay awake and mentally alert. Useful when driving, studying, doing repetitive tasks, or when you need to be alert. Great as a mid-morning or afternoon pick-me-up. Contains no caffeine, sugar or stimulants. Does not cause jitters.

How it works: Supports mental clarity, physical energy, adrenal gland function and blood circulation.

Herbal

Ingredients: Asian Kirin red Ginseng root, Fo-ti cured root, Gotu Kola herb, Siberian Eleuthero root, Damiana leaf, cultivated American Ginseng root, Licorice root, Prickly Ash bark, fresh Peppermint herb, Ginger root and Cayenne fruit.

Suggested Use: Take one softgel or 30 drops with water mid-morning, mid-afternoon or as needed as a natural, quick pick-me-up.

Contraindications: Do not use during pregnancy.

Yeast *ReLeaf*®

What it's for: **Internally**: Use for intestinal or systemic candida infection with resulting irregularities: diarrhea or constipation, bloating, low or fluctuating energy levels, vaginitis, menstrual difficulties, and/or allergic reactions to foods. Also used for thrush or mouth fungal infection, sinus infection, and certain types of eczema aggravated by candida. **Externally**: Useful on athlete's foot.

How it works: Supports a healthy intestinal and vaginal tract. Promotes internal cleansing. Assists the body in maintaining proper levels of *Candida albicans* within the intestinal tract. Inhibits fungal growth.

Ingredients: Pau D'Arco inner bark, Quassia inner wood, Licorice root, *Echinacea angustifolia* root, Myrrh gum resin, Yerba Mansa root, fresh Black "green" walnut hull (tree-nut), fresh Thuja leaf, Astragalus root and fresh Garlic clove.

Suggested Use: **Internally**: Take one softgel or 30 drops with water three to four times a day. **Externally**: One teaspoon of the extract in a half cup of boiled water. Douche or apply when water cools. (For douche, add 1/8 teaspoon salt to the boiled water.)

Contraindications: Do not use during pregnancy.

CHAPTER 8

Used in Formulas

...the herbs found in formulas featured in the Herbal Directory (Chapter 7).

Note that when an herb is designated as a "fresh herb", it means the herb has not been dried prior to extraction. The herb is extracted while fresh and succulent. You will find suggested use recommendations, possible contraindications, side effects, and/or warnings under each specific formula.

Information on single herbs found in formulas

Andrographis
(*Andrographis paniculata,* dried herb) Ideal herb for the first day of a cold or flu. Specific for early colds and flu, acute and chronic infections, pharyngolaryngitis, cough with thick mucus, and weakened immune system. Protects the liver against the effects of alcohol, aspirin, acetaminophen, NSAIDS (non-steroidal anti-inflammatory drugs) or other known liver-toxic substances. Great support in poor liver function. Helpful in worm infestations, diarrhea, and dysentery. Also useful in skin abscesses and sores. Protects sinus, throat and lung tissues. Supports and enhances healthy liver function in a manner similar to Milk Thistle. In combination with acidophilus, restores healthy intestinal environment.

Angelica
(*Angelica archangelica,* root) Stimulates gastric secretions, stops flatulence, helpful in nervous stomach, rheumatic and skin disorders.

Ashwagandha
(*Withania somnifera,* dried root) Useful for debility, nervous exhaustion especially due to stress or acute illness, emaciation, convalescence, chronic disease especially if inflammatory in nature, e.g. connective-tissue disease, rheumatoid and osteoarthritis, general tonic and depressed white blood cell count. Possesses significant adaptogenic effects. Increases stress endurance

Single Herbs Used in Formulas 87

and prevents stress-induced effects on entire body. Demonstrates strong immunomodulatory and anti-inflammatory properties.

Astragalus
(*Astragalus membranaceus* [huang qi], dried root) Useful for people with frequent or chronic infectious diseases such as bronchitis, sinusitis, hepatitis B, and chronic non-healing sores. Useful for people who are debilitated, lacking in energy or vitality. Helpful for individuals who are unable to withstand or feel vulnerable when faced with increased stress. Counteracts the immune system suppression associated with cancer therapy.

Balsam poplar
(*Populus balsamifera,* bud) Also known as Balm of Gilead. Stimulates expectoration, helps liquefy mucus.

Bayberry
(*Morella pensylvanica,* root bark). For chronic inflammation of mouth, gastrointestinal tract and respiratory system, bleeding gums and sore throat. For diarrhea from stress or excess food;, for colitis or dysentery.

Bethroot
(*Trillium erectum,* root) Eases irregular menstrual periods, menstrual pain and excessive vaginal discharge. Decreases inflammatory prostaglandin production in reproductive tissues. Aids childbirth.

Betony
(*Pedicularis canadensis,* fresh herb) Quiets anxieties, tension and hyperactive states. Relaxes skeletal muscles.

Black cherry
(*Prunus serotina,* bark) Useful for coughs and bronchial congestion.

Black cohosh
(*Actaea racemosa,* dried root) Useful for menopausal women experiencing hot flashes, thinning and drying of vaginal lining, night sweats and mild depression. For dull aching pains (without acute inflammation) of joints, muscles or uterus.

Use in conjunction with Blue Cohosh as a traditional support during labor and for the after-birth (postpartum) period. Promotes a healthy estrogen to progesterone balance. Supports healthy joints, muscles and related connective tissues in post-menopausal women. Strengthens weak, irregular uterine contractions during labor. Decreases after-birth pains.

Black currant
(*Ribes nigrum,* fresh leaf) Supports weak adrenal glands. Enhances adrenal gland health.

Black haw
(*Viburnum prunifolium,* stem bark) Useful for painful menstruation. Especially sharp, stabbing-like cramps. Calms uterine contractions. Prevents miscarriages.

Black walnut
(*Juglans nigra,* fresh green hull) Promotes healthy skin and intestines. Supports beneficial bacterial flora in the intestines by preventing and stopping the overgrowth of fungus.
Supports healthy skin, mouth, throat, stomach, intestines and vagina.

Bloodroot
(*Sanguinaria canadensis,* root) Stops coughs. Prevents plaque buildup on teeth.

Blue flag
(*Iris versicolor,* root) Stimulates production of pancreatic enzymes and bile. Useful in skin eruptions from high stress and poor diet. Stimulates saliva and sweat secretions.

Boldo
(*Peumus boldus,* leaf) Stimulates bile secretion. Eases constipation, digestive disorders and liver insufficiencies. Inhibits urinary bacterial infections.

Buchu
(*Agathosma betulina,* leaf) Decreases kidney inflammation. Stops urinary tract infections.

Burdock
(*Arctium lappa,* root) Effective in dry and scaly eczema, psoriasis, acne, dandruff and boils.

Supports healthy skin moisture levels when dry and scaly. Helps skin and scalp retain their elasticity. Stimulates digestive juices, bile secretion and excretion of urea and uric acid.

Calendula
(*Calendula officinalis,* flower) **Internally:** Stimulates immune system function. For inflammation of the mouth and peptic ulcers. **Externally:** Heals skin burns or inflammation, abrasions, pressure ulcers (i.e., bedsores), and impetigo (also see Usnea).

California poppy
(*Eschscholzia californica,* fresh flowering plant) Specific for people who have difficulty staying asleep or who wake up too early in the morning. Permits deep sleep. Great for sleepless, frenetic children or for children who sleep so soundly that they wet the bed. Ensures ongoing sleep during the night. Balances sleep depth.

California spikenard
(*Aralia californica,* root) Decreases perception and effects of stress. Although most adaptogens originate from the Orient, this one comes from the Amercian west coast.

Cardamom
(*Elettaria cardamomum,* seed) Soothes stomach lining, decreases stomach and pelvic cramps. Reduces intestinal gas production.

Cassia
(*Cinnamomum aromaticum* [gui zhi], twig) Lowers elevated body temperature and induces perspiration.

Catnip
(*Nepeta cataria,* flower top) Calms frenetic children. Taken hot, stimulates sweating in colds and flu, and breaks up fevers. Taken cold, eases stomach and intestinal cramps in adults and especially in children.

Cayenne
(*Capsicum annuum,* dried fruit) During viral infections, it cools dry, hot mucous membranes. Useful in cases of dry mouth or a lack of digestive secretions due to nervousness, alcohol

abuse, prescription drugs and old age. Useful in poor peripheral circulation with cold hands and feet.

Celandine
(*Chelidonium majus,* herb) Protects liver from injury. Decreases gastrointestinal cramping. Stimulates bile flow.

Chamomile
(*Matricaria recutita,* whole fresh flower) Useful for mild anxiety, sleep problems, mild indigestion, flatulence, mild gastritis, gingivitis, mucositis, gastrointestinal upsets and menstrual-related migraines. Supports healthy nervous system. Maintains healthy inflammatory response of the digestive system. Reduces mild skin inflammation and supports skin rejuvenation. **Externally:** For skin inflammation, atopic eczema and skin irritation.

Chaste tree
See Vitex

Chinese lovage
(*Ligusticum jeholense* [liao gao ben], root) Relieves congestion, dampness and headaches.

Chinese mint
(*Mentha canadensis* [bo he], herb) Useful for headaches, fever, lack of perspiration, dry mouth and/or throat.

Chinese rhubarb
(*Rheum officinal* [da huang], root) Laxative with astringent properties. Small amounts balance the intestinal function. Useful for either constipation, traveler's diarrhea or chronic diarrhea.

Cinnamon
(*Cinnamomum verum,* dried bark) Useful for elevated blood sugar, abdominal bloating, gas, mild intestinal cramps and diarrhea. Curbs excessive menstrual bleeding. Helps maintain healthy blood sugar and triglyceride levels. Stimulates digestion and protects stomach tissues. Enhances normal blood coagulation and healthy blood vessel tone in lungs and uterus.

Cleavers
(*Galium aparine,* herb) Stimulates lymphatic drainage especially of the pelvic area. Useful for urinary tract and skin problems. Supports elimination of waste products through the lymphatic system, liver and kidneys.

Clove
(*Syzygium aromaticum,* flower bud) Possesses antispasmodic properties. Relieves menstrual cramps, nausea, and vomiting.

Cordyceps
(*Cordyceps hawkesii,* [dong chong xia cao], mycelium) Adaptogen (i.e., a substance that produces a normalizing effect on the body). Increases resistance to stress and infection. Supports lung and reproductive functions.

Couch grass
(*Elymus repens,* root) Effective diuretic. Increases elimination of urinary waste products.

Cramp bark
(*Viburnum opulus,* bark) Specific for acute menstrual cramps where symptoms include strong, sharp, stabbing-like pains.

Cranberry
(*Vaccinium macrocarpon,* fruit) Prevent adhesion of bacteria (especially E. coli) to bladder wall epithelial cells. Decreases incidence of and prevents urinary tract infections.

Cubeb
(*Piper cubeba,* berry) Inhibits bacterial growth in sinus, respiratory and urinary tract.

Culver's root
(*Veronicastrum virginicum,* root) Stimulates production of bile. Promotes the health function of the liver.

Damiana
(*Turnera diffusa,* leaf) Useful for anxiety and depression. Use for irritation of urinary tissues and reproductive tissues (urethra, bladder and vagina) caused by emotional stress, sexual tension or stress due to traveling. Useful in delayed menstruation in young girls. Has a reputation as an aphrodisiac.

Dandelion
(*Taraxacum officinale,* root) For poor bile secretion, poor appetite and digestive function, constipation from lack of bile, rheumatic conditions, eczema, chronic skin eruptions, or psoriasis aggravated by emotional stress and/or fatty foods. Supports healthy liver and gallbladder functions. Stimulates digestive function and proper elimination of waste products through the liver and intestines. Promotes healthy skin.

Devil's claw
(*Harpagophytum procumbens,* storage tuber) Safe anti-inflammatory for arthritis, rheumatism, gout, joint inflammation, gallbladder problems with pancreatic distress, and for elevated cholesterol and uric acid blood levels.

Dong quai
(*Angelica sinensis* [dang qui], cured root slice) For menopausal challenges. For PMS with dull, aching pain before or during menstruation. In deficient estrogen or testosterone secretion, it increases cellular uptake of these hormones in uterine, vaginal, ovarian or prostatic tissues.

Echinacea angustifolia
(*Echinacea angustifolia*, dried root)
A must in the beginning stages of a cold or flu. Excellent for tendonitis, bursitis, tennis elbow, skier's knee and jogger's ankle. Gets rid of dead microbes, dead cells and other lymphatic waste products. **Externally:** Effective on swollen areas due to bee, wasp, gnat and mosquito bites.

Echinacea pallida
(*Echinacea pallida,* root) Similar properties as Echinacea angustifolia.

Echinacea purpurea
(*Echinacea purpurea,* herb, root & flower) Similar properties as *Echinacea angustifolia*.

Elder: berry
(*Sambucus nigra*, fresh berry) Taken in the early stages of flu, it prevents the virus from taking hold. Used traditionally as a spring cleanser.

Elder: flower (*Sambucus nigra,* fresh flower)
Induces sweating and reduces fever during flu/colds or fevers.

Single Herbs Used in Formulas

Elecampane
(*Inula helenium*, root) Useful for chronic coughs, allergies, asthma and lung infections. Relieves bronchial spasms.

Eleuthero, Siberian
(formerly Siberian Ginseng)
(*Eleutherococcus senticosus*, dried root) Not a true "Panax" ginseng, but has similar actions. Increases endurance and resistance to stress or infection. Helpful for those who thrive on stress (type *A* personalities). An excellent adaptogen (i.e.: a substance that produces a normalizing effect on the body). Can be taken for extended periods of time.

European mistletoe
(*Viscum album*, leaf twig) Helps reduce elevated blood pressure.

Eyebright
(*Euphrasia rostkoviana*, dried herb) Take for hay fever and allergies with watery eyes, sneezing, runny nose, frontal headache and stuffy sinuses. In diluted form, use externally for redness and swelling in cases of conjunctivitis or blepharitis. Calms fixed antibodies located in eyes, sinus, nose and respiratory tissues. Acts as a mild astringent on mucous membranes.

Fennel
(*Foeniculum vulgare*, seed) Reduces inflammation and relieves stomach and intestinal gas. Decreases dyspepsia and diarrhea in infants. Use externally for conjunctivitis or blepharitis.

Feverfew
(*Tanacetum parthenium*, herb) Useful to prevent and treat migraine headaches (reduces severity and frequency of attacks). Possesses anti-inflammatory properties. Helpful in psoriasis and arthritis.

Fo-ti
(*Polygonum multiflorum* [he shou wu], cured root) Possesses tonifying and rejuvenating properties. Decreases insomnia, constipation and atherosclerosis.

Fringe tree
(*Chionanthus virginicus*, root bark) Relieves congestion of the liver. Increases excretion of bile. Aids digestion. Promotes assimilation of nutrients.

Garlic
(*Allium sativum,* clove) Has significant antibacterial and antiviral properties. Use for colds, flu, bronchitis, rhinitis, bacterial, viral and fungal infections, high cholesterol and hypertension.

Gentian
(*Gentiana lutea,* root) Improves and strengthens digestion. Stimulates appetite.

Ginger
(*Zingiber officinale,* dried root) Relieves motion sickness; works better than Dramamine® for chemotherapy, postoperative, pregnancy-related, or vertigo nausea as well as vomiting. Relieves indigestion, abdominal and menstrual cramping, dyspepsia and gastric hypoacidity. Useful in acute colds and flu. Supports healthy digestion. Enhances gastrointestinal transport. Also calms vomiting centers in the brain. Induces sweating during dry fevers.

Ginkgo
(*Ginkgo biloba,* fresh leaf) Use for hearing and sight disorders from poor blood flow in ears and eyes. Helpful for Alzheimer's disease, vertigo associated with inner-ear problems, tinnitus, loss of memory and alertness. For poor circulation problems in eyes, skin, and extremities when diabetes is present. Supports healthy blood circulation to the brain, ears, eyes, skin and extremities. Has a scavenging effect on free radicals and exerts anti-stress actions. Improves memory, concentration and moods.

Ginseng, American cultivated
(*Panax quinquefolius* [xi yang shen], root) Mildest of the American ginsengs. Same indications as Ginseng, American wild.

Ginseng, American wild
(*Panax quinquefolius* [xi yang shen], root) Strongest American ginseng. Excellent adaptogen and long-term tonic. Strengthens the mind. Use in mild depression, chronic fatigue syndrome, fibromyalgia, chronic stress and in post performance immune depletion in athletes. Useful in menopause when other menopausal herbs don't seem to work. Also increases vaginal moistness during menopause.

Single Herbs Used in Formulas 95

Ginseng, American woodsgrown
(*Panax quinquefolius* [xi yang shen], root) This ginseng is stronger than American cultivated but weaker than American wild Ginseng. To learn its indications see Ginseng, American wild.

Ginseng, Asian red Kirin
(*Panax ginseng,* [ren shen] cured dried root) Most stimulating of the ginsengs. Identical to Asian red Shui Chu except that it comes from a different province in China. For physical or emotional stress or exhaustion, mild depression and tiredness. Useful for older people whose appetite, energy and stamina are low, especially while recuperating from disease or surgery. As an adaptogen (i.e., a substance that produces a normalizing effect on the body) it exerts a strengthening effect and raises physical and mental capacity. Increases resistance to the negative effects of physical, chemical or biological stress.

Ginseng, Asian white
(*Panax ginseng,* dried root) [ren shen] Considered stronger than Siberian Eleuthero but weaker than American Ginseng. For emotional and physical stress manifesting as elevated blood sugar, cholesterol and triglycerides as well as exhaustion and depression. Use when recuperating from illness or surgery. For emotional and physical well being. An excellent adaptogen (i.e., a substance that produces a normalizing effect on the body), it increases endurance, and resistance to stress or infection. Maintains stamina and positive mental outlook.

Goldenseal
(*Hydrastis canadensis,* dried root and rhizome) Use for a subacute or chronic mucous membrane inflammation occurring in sinusitis, hay fever, allergies, gastritis, stomach ulcers, colitis, sore gums and throat, diarrhea or tonsillitis.

Gotu kola
(*Centella asiatica,* dried herb) Specific for low thyroid gland function contributing to emotional depression, dry skin, cold extremities, poor digestion, weight gain and/or low endurance. Use also for eczema, psoriasis and varicose veins. Supports thyroid gland. Contributes to emotional health, skin health, warm extremities,

healthy digestion, healthy weight and/or increased endurance. Enhances memory, clarity and calmness. Supports healthy connective tissue of the veins' vascular walls. Research supports its use to increase the collagen content of challenged skin and promotes healthy wound healing.

Grindelia
(*Grindelia camporum* et al. flower) Specific for thick and hard-to-move mucus, harsh and dry coughs and difficulty breathing due to congestion. Specific for dermatitis caused by poison ivy or oak. Useful for chronic skin ulcers to accelerate healing.

Hawthorn
(*Crataegus* spp., fresh berry, dried leaf, and flower) For mild heart irregularities with rapid heartbeat episodes or weakness of heart muscle from poor coronary blood supply and mild angina.

Holy Basil
(*Ocimum tenuiflorum*, dried leaf of Krishna and Rama Tulsi) First-class adaptogen. Excellent in high stress situations. It increases overall resistance. Supports a healthy immune system. Keeps blood sugar levels, blood pressure, and cholesterol and triglycerides in the healthy range. Protects against the side effects of radio- and chemotherapy.

Honeysuckle
(*Lonicera* spp. [jin yin hua], flower) Use for common cold and influenza. Prevents upper respiratory tract infections.

Hops
(*Humulus lupulus*, strobile) Useful for insomnia, restlessness, stress-related tension and anxiety. Specific against Gram-positive bacterial infections (staph, strep, pneumococcus).

Horehound
(*Marrubium vulgare*, herb) Use for coughs, colds and lung problems. A warm tea of the extract will produce diaphoresis (sweating).

Horsetail
(*Equisetum arvense*, herb) Useful for children who

Single Herbs Used in Formulas 97

wet the bed. Stimulates intestinal calcium absorption. Strengthens connective tissue weakness, especially of the lungs, joints and urinary tract.

Jack-in-the-pulpit
(*Arisaema triphyllum,* tuber) Specific for sore throats, excessive talking, screaming, shouting, hoarseness and loss of voice.

Jamaica dogwood
(*Piscidia piscipula,* bark) Reduces muscular and nervous system pain.

Jewel weed
(*Impatiens capensis,* herb) Specific for poison ivy, poison oak, stinging nettle, hives, mullein rash and other types of dermatitis (skin inflammation) caused by plant contact.

Juniper
(*Juniperus communis,* berry) Useful as an antiseptic in subacute or chronic inflammation of the bladder or urethra. Also for chronic arthritis, gout and rheumatism.

Kava
(*Piper methysticum*, dried root) Relieves nervousness, agitation, tension, stress and anxiety. Relaxes muscle tension due to stress, relieves fatigue and calms the mind. Useful when anxiety prevents sleep.

Lavender
(*Lavandula angustifolia,* flower) Relieves abdominal bloating, intestinal or stomach gas and indigestion. Calms and settles the restless person.

Lemon balm
(*Melissa officinalis,* herb) Relieves nervousness, insomnia, nausea, digestive disturbances and anxiety. Used externally and internally to relieve herpes simplex cold sores.

Lesser periwinkle
(*Vinca minor,* herb) Useful for headaches, vertigo, memory loss and difficulty in remembering. Increases cerebral blood flow.

Licorice
(*Glycyrrhiza glabra,* dried root) For gastric ulcers, bronchial spasms, sore throats, painful

menstruation, arthritis or herpes. Inhibits viral replication; although the inhibiting mechanism of action has not been discovered yet. Supports healthy adrenal gland function. Maintains healthy gastric and duodenal linings. Soothes the throat and bronchioles. Supports healthy inflammatory response. Possesses intestinal regulating effects.

Linden
(*Tilia cordata*, flower) Induces sweating in colds and infections, reduces nasal congestion, relieves throat irritation in cough. Used to treat nervous palpitations and relieve high blood pressure.

Lobelia
(*Lobelia inflata*, fresh herb in bladder seed stage) Specific for bronchial spasms that may occur in asthma. Binds to nicotine receptor sites in the body, thus decreasing nicotine cravings. Maintains healthy bronchial tone. Enhances lung mucus expectoration.

Lomatium
(*Lomatium dissectum*, root) Use for influenza, lung problems, head colds, fevers, pneumonia and persistent winter fevers.

Magnolia
(*Magnolia acuminate* [xin yi hua], bud) Unblocks nasal obstruction, relieves sinusitis and rhinitis.

Maitake
(*Grifola frondosa*, fruiting body) Possesses adaptogenic properties. Useful to treat diabetes, high blood pressure and high cholesterol. Excellent support during chemo or radiation therapy as it decreases side effects from these treatments.

Male fern
(*Dryopteris filix-mas*, root) Traditional medicine for the treatment of parasites.

Meadowsweet
(*Filipendula ulmaria*, herb) Reduces acid indigestion, gastritis and peptic ulcers. Decreases inflammation in rheumatic, arthritic or urinary disorders

Single Herbs Used in Formulas 99

Milk Thistle
(*Silybum marianum,* dried seed) <u>The premier liver herb</u>. Useful for chronic hepatitis, fatty liver of alcoholics, or cirrhosis of the liver. Use when exposed to harmful substances such as alcohol, fumes and drugs. Protects individuals who have had long-term exposure to chemicals, metals or aromatic hydro-carbons, such as solvents, paints, thinner, etc.

Motherwort
(*Leonurus cardiaca,* herb) Calms rapid heartbeat, palpitation and hypertension from thyroid stress. Restores elasticity and secretion of postmenopausal vaginal walls. Decreases frequency and severity of hot flashes.

Mullein
(*Verbascum thapsus,* fresh leaf) Specific for coughs, especially in older asthmatic individuals. Useful for subacute or chronic bronchitis, emphysema or chronic obstructive pulmonary disease which worsens with nervousness. Offers support in ongoing lung and throat challenges. Relaxes bronchial spasms. Acts as mild lung sedative.

Myrrh
(*Commiphora myrrha,* gum exudate) For painful ulceration of the gums or mouth experience in herpes or gingivitis. Useful in pharyngitis, sinusitis, laryngitis and indigestion. Taken in combination with Echinacea, Myrrh helps to elevate low white blood cell levels. Promotes healthy gums and oral tissues. Possesses astringent properties on mucous membranes.

Oat
(*Avena sativa,* fresh seed in milky stage) Nervous system tonic. Use in nervous exhaustion, edginess, emotional breakdown and for the person who wishes to withdraw from nicotine, cocaine or opiates.

Ocotillo
(*Fouquieria splendens,* stem) Relieves lymphatic and venous congestion. Relieves pelvic congestion, hemorrhoids, benign prostate enlargements and cervical varicosities. Stimulates lymph drainage.

Olive
(*Olea europaea*, dried leaf) Helpful in the beginning of bacterial, viral and fungal infections. Use for colds and flu, upper-respiratory infection, ear infection and sinusitis. For mildly to moderate elevated blood pressure. Reduces the severity and healing time of herpes outbreaks.

Orange
(*Citrus sinensis,* peel) In Chinese medicine, used to enhance the function of other herbs.

Oregon grape
(*Mahonia aquifolium,* root) A good bitter tonic. Helps resolve indigestion and poor appetite. Stimulates digestion, absorption, and assimilation. Use in acne, psoriasis, herpes flare-ups, eczema and any other skin conditions, especially when constipation is present. Also useful in parasitic infection, especially giardia. Possesses antibacterial activity.

Osha
(*Ligusticum porteri,* dried root)
Supportive herb at the beginning of a cold or flu. For sore throat, chest cold with painful breathing, thick stringy mucus or dry asthma. Prevents recurrent middle-ear infections in children.

Parsley
(*Petroselinum crispum,* root) A simple, effective diuretic.

Passionflower
(*Passiflora incarnata*, fresh herb tip) For the "chattering" brain which prevents sleep. Calms the mind in headstrong individuals. Good for menopausal nervousness and anxiety, for moderately elevated blood pressure and for persistent hiccup.

Pau d'arco
(*Tabebuia impetiginosa,* Argentinian dried inner bark) **Internally:** Take for systemic *Candida albicans* infection, and fungal infections of the mouth (thrush). It supports proper flora balance for the intestines and vagina and assists the body in maintaining proper levels of *Candida*

albicans. **Externally:** Use for fungal infection in feet, babies' bottoms or women's vaginas. Offers potent antifungal action.

Pelargonium
(*Pelargonium sidoides* [umckaloabo], dried root) Useful for sinus, tonsils, throat, and lung infections, acute bronchitis, coughs and mucus accumulation in the lungs. Useful for children with respiratory infections who are not responding well or not getting better with repeated antibiotic treatments. Provides rapid respiratory immune system stimulation. Prevents viral invasion of respiratory cells. Prevents bacteria from attaching to mucous membrane cells. Enhances interferon production and activation of natural killer cells. Increases cilia (hair-like projections) movements in lungs and stimulates mucus removal.

Peppermint
(*Mentha piperita,* fresh herb) Stops stomach and intestinal cramping, ingestion and nausea. Calms stomach and soothes the smooth muscles of the gastrointestinal tract. Stimulates the production and release of bile. Prevents intestinal fermentation and stops gas formation.

Pipsissewa
(*Chimaphila umbellata,* herb) For bladder, kidney or urethra irritation or infection. Helps prevent recurring urinary tract infection. Use for prostate irritation when dull pain occurs after the first morning urination. Eliminates waste products.

Plantain
(*Plantago major,* leaf) Decreases inflammation and speeds healing of surface tissues including sinuses, bronchioles, stomach and skin.

Pleurisy root
(*Asclepias tuberosa,* root) Useful in pleurisy, pneumonia, bronchitis or chest colds with dry respiratory membranes and skin. For dry skin problems, such as eczema or psoriasis.

Prickly ash
(*Zanthoxylum americanum,* bark) Tones mucous tissues and decreases excessive secretions. Stimulates sluggish circulation especially to the extremities and brain tissues.

Propolis
(Dry gum from beehives) **Internally:** For mouth, gum and intestinal infections; foul-smelling diarrhea from intestinal infections. Balances harmful and beneficial inflammatory compounds. Supports healthy intestinal membrane function during dietary and microbial challenges. **Externally:** For skin abrasions, especially in moist areas such as feet, hands and face. Supports healthy skin.

Quassia
(*Quassia amara,* inner wood) Classic remedy to eliminate worms and yeast from the bowels. Excellent bitter to aid digestion.

Red root
(*Ceanothus americanus,* root) For acute tonsillitis or sore throat; inflamed spleen and/or inflamed lymphatic nodes, and fluid-filled cysts in breasts, ovaries, uterus or testes. Supports healthy lymphatic system. Stimulates fluid drainage from congested tissues. Supports drainage of uterine, ovarian, breast or testicular tissues.

Reishi
(*Ganoderma lucidum* [ling zhi], fruiting body) Adaptogen. Long-term immune and nervous system tonic. Protects and enhances the internal organ functions: heart, liver, kidneys, nervous system, reproductive system, lungs, stomach and adrenal glands. Decreases allergic reactions and offers support during cancer, chemotherapy or radiation therapy.

Rosemary
(*Rosmarinus officinalis,* leaf) Supports liver and gallbladder function. Decreases gastrointestinal upset, gas and bloating. Improves circulation and memory. Acts as a mild mood elevator.

Sarsaparilla
(*Smilax febrifuga,* root) Increases elimination of urea and uric acid. Helpful in gout, herpes, skin problems, rheumatism and sores. For moderate deficiencies of adrenal or gonad hormonal production. Useful in benign prostate enlargement.

Saw palmetto
(*Serenoa repens,* dried berry) Specific for simple prostate enlargement, difficulty urinating, especially with benign prostatic hypertrophy and dribbling of urine. Supports healthy prostate function. Contributes to normal urination. Helps balance harmful and beneficial inflammatory compounds in these tissues and increases uptake of circulating male hormones.

Schisandra
(*Schisandra chinensis* [wu wei zi], berry) Increases overall resistance. Supports healthy adrenal and liver function. Helps fight stress, fatigue, tiredness, exhaustion and depression. Use for allergic skin disorders. Considered nearly as good as ginseng.

Sheep sorrel
(*Rumex acetosella,* herb) Increases excretion of waste products.

Shiitake
(*Lentinula edodes* [siang xun], fruiting body) Regulates the immune system. Use for chronic fatigue syndrome, candida overgrowth, allergies, Herpes Simplex I and II, frequent colds and bronchitis. Protects the liver. Lowers cholesterol and blood lipids. Offers support for HIV, during cancer, chemotherapy or radiation therapy.

Skullcap
(*Scutellaria lateriflora,* fresh flowering herb) For inability to sleep, edgy feelings, restlessness, phantom pains after amputation, muscle twitches, neuralgia, pain from shingles, and sciatica. Soothes and strengthens the peripheral nervous system which is ultimately involved with the skin and the five senses: sight, sound, smell, taste and touch.

Slippery elm
(*Ulmus rubra,* dried inner bark) Useful for gastritis, enteritis, colitis, mouth and throat inflammation, duodenal ulcers, and diarrhea. Soothes, protects and heals mucous membranes of the mouth, throat, bronchioles, stomach, intestines and duodenum. Regulates intestinal function, useful for both diarrhea and constipation.

Spikenard
(*Aralia racemosa,* root) Use for coughs and irritation of the lungs especially when excessive mucus is present.

Spilanthes
(*Spilanthes oleracea,* herb) Similar immunostimulating and lymphatic properties as Echinacea. Useful for colds, flu or when the immune system is challenged.

St. John's wort
(*Hypericum perforatum,* fresh and dry flower in the bud stage) Acts as a natural mood elevator and supports emotional stability. Offers support during mild to moderate depression, anxiety, agitation, insomnia, loss of interest, and excessive sleeping. Calms nerve pain from crushed or cut nerves, hitting your thumb with a hammer or slamming your finger in the car door. Calms irritated nerve fibers.

Star anise
(*Illcium verum,* fruit) Useful for abdominal pain, gas and bloating.

Stevia
(*Stevia rebaudiana,* herb) Use as a sweetening agent. Normalizes blood pressure and regulates the heartbeat.

Stillingia
(*Stillingia sylvatica,* root) Supports the elimination of waste products by the lymphatic system.

Stinging nettle
(*Urtica dioica,* fresh herb) Contains high levels of chlorophyll. Specific for hay fever and allergic rhinitis. Also for vaginitis, rheumatoid arthritis, stomatitis, eczema, diarrhea, hemorrhoids, asthma and gout caused by allergies. Useful for mucous membranes especially where excessive mucus and inflammation are present. Stabilizes mast-cell walls and fixed antibodies found in the eyes and respiratory system, keeping the tissues calm. Tones mucous membranes. An alkalizing diuretic.

Stoneroot
(*Collinsonia canadensis,* fresh root) Excellent herb for laryngitis, pharyngitis, loss of voice and other throat challenges.

Single Herbs Used in Formulas

Thuja
(*Thuja occidentalis,* leaf) Useful against candida and other intestinal fungi.

Toadflax
(*Linaria vulgaris,* herb) Stimulates the processing of liver waste products by specialized liver cells called Kupffer cells. Normalizes production of liver enzymes. Use in chronic liver inflammation and hepatitis flare-ups.

Turmeric
(*Curcuma longa*) Delivers strong anti-inflammatory activity in acute and chronic allergies. It stops the production of inflammatory compounds that create havoc in the respiratory and digestive tissues.

Usnea
(*Usnea barbata*, dried lichen) **Internally:** Specific for pneumonia, pleurisy, bronchitis, sinusitis, cystitis, urethritis, sore and/or strep throat caused by bacterial infections. **Externally:** Use for staph, strep or fungal infection, impetigo, athlete's foot, ringworm, abrasions and skin irritations or as a douche in trichomonas infection. Supports mouth, gum, stomach and intestinal mucous membranes. Works in a similar way to Goldenseal. Strengthens respiratory tissues including sinus, throat, lungs and bronchioles. Inhibits Gram-positive bacterial microorganisms. Protects and heals skin.

Uva-ursi
(*Arctostaphylos uva-ursi,* leaf) Possesses significant antibacterial and anti-inflammatory activities especially in urinary tract infections. May prevent kidney stone formation.

Valerian
(*Valeriana officinalis,* fresh root) Use for insomnia, emotional depression, poor sleep from pain or trauma, and gastrointestinal or uterine cramps, especially in the weakened person. For nervousness, anxiety, and stress-related hypertension.

Vitex
(*Vitex agnus-castus* [Chaste Tree], dried berry) For premenstrual syndrome (PMS), painful breasts, vaginal dryness, low libido, mild depression, menopausal changes, acne and premenstrual herpes on the lips. Stimulates milk production in nursing mothers.

White pine
(*Vitex agnus-castus* [Chaste Tree], dried berry) For premenstrual syndrome (PMS), painful breasts, vaginal dryness, low libido, mild depression, menopausal changes, acne and premenstrual herpes on the lips. Stimulates milk production in nursing mothers.

White pine
(*Pinus strobus,* bark) Calms cough and throat irritations.

White willow
(*Salix alba,* bark) Useful for headache, fevers, inflammation of joints and membranes, muscle aches, gout, bursitis and tendonitis.

Wild indigo
(*Baptisia tinctoria,* root) Specific for ulcerations of mucous membranes of the mouth, stomach and intestines. Strong lymphatic stimulant. Eliminates waste products.

Wild yam
(*Dioscorea villosa,* fresh root) Helps stop cramps or spasms of "hollow organs," such as intestines, gall bladder, uterus, bladder and ureters. Relieves inflammation in acute rheumatoid arthritis, and diverticulosis. Excellent for morning sickness. Helps ease stomach or intestinal irritability after operations. Decreases nervous system impulses to the muscular walls of hollow organs. Acts as an anti-inflammatory.

Witch hazel
(*Hamamelis virginiana,* bark) Use for poor venous drainage when veins are dilated, excessively relaxed, enlarged and full. Helpful with varicose veins, hemorrhoids, spongy gums, phlebitis and diarrhea.

Wormwood
(*Artemisia absinthium,* herb) Effective against protozoa and giardia.

Xanthium
(*Xanthium sibiricum* [cang er zi], fruit) Opens nasal passages and relieves pain. Use for sinusitis, rhinitis, sinus headaches, nasal blockage or loss of smell.

Yarrow
(*Achillea millefolium,* flower top) Effective in the early stages of colds or flu with fever. Decreases inflammation of reproductive and urinary tract mucous membranes.

Yellow dock
(*Rumex crispus,* root) Useful for constipation, blood disorders, skin diseases, liver congestion, poor digestion of fatty foods, jaundice and post-hepatitis flare-ups. Helps increase iron absorption in digestive tract.

Yerba mansa
(*Anemopsis californica,* root) Possesses an action similar to Goldenseal. Reduces inflammation of skin and mucous membranes. Use for sinus, mouth, gum, throat, lung, stomach, intestinal, bladder and vaginal inflammation. Also contains antibacterial and antifungal properties.

Yerba santa
(*Eriodictyon californicum,* leaf) Specific for thin, watery, dripping mucus from hayfever, colds, allergies or other sinus and lung problems.

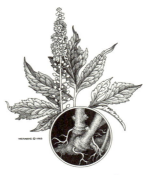

Black Cohosh

CHAPTER 9

Health Condition Index

Notes on this Health Condition Index

This index cross-references recommended herbal formulas for health conditions listed in alphabetical order from A (Abdominal pain) to Y (Yeast infection). For detailed information on each suggested synergistic formula or single herb, consult the **Herbal Directory** (Chapter 7).

Abdominal pain
Stomach Tonic™

Abrasions, skin
Phytocillin® (internally & extenally)

Abscess
Lymphatonic™
Phytocillin®

Adaptogen
Deep Health®
Stress *ReLeaf*®
Ultimate Ginseng™

Addiction
Adrenotonic™

Adrenal support
Adrenotonic™

Agitation
Kava Cool Complex™
Nervine Tonic™

Alcoholism
Liver Tonic™

Alertness
Ultimate Ginseng™
Vibrant Energy™

Allergic rhinitis
Allergy *ReLeaf*® System
Allertonic®

Allergic skin disorders
Allergy *ReLeaf*® System
Allertonic®

Allergies, acute
Allergy *ReLeaf*® System
Allertonic®

Allergies, prevention of
Adrenotonic™
Allergy *ReLeaf*® System
Allertonic®
Deep Health®

Altitude acclimation
ChlorOxygen®

Anemia
ChlorOxygen®

Antihistamine
Allergy *ReLeaf*® System
Allertonic®

Anxiety
Kava Cool Complex™
Nervine Tonic™
Stress *ReLeaf*®

Arthritis, acute pain from
Herbaprofen®

Asthma, acute
Congest Free™

Asthma, chronic
Adrenotonic™
Allergy *ReLeaf*® System
Lung Tonic™

Athlete's foot
ParaFree™ (externally & internally)
Yeast *ReLeaf*® (externally)

Health Condition Index

Autoimmune disorders
Adrenotonic™
Deep Health®
Essiac Tonic

Back pain
Herbaprofen®

Bacterial infection
Loviral™
Peak Defense™
Phytocillin®

Bartholin gland cyst
Lymphatonic™

Bedsores
Lymphatonic™
Phytocillin® (externally)

Bell's palsy
Nervine Tonic™
Stress *ReLeaf*®

Bile secretion
Liver Tonic™

Bilirubin, high levels of
Liver Tonic™

Birth pains
Cramp *ReLeaf*®

Bites, bug
Bug Itch *ReLeaf*® (externally)
Echinacea Triple Source™ (externally & internally)
Ivy Itch ReLeaf® (externally)

Bladder irritation or infection
CranBladder *ReLeaf*®
Kidney Tonic™

Bloating
ParaFree™
Stomach Tonic™
Yeast *ReLeaf*®

Blood builder
ChlorOxygen®

Blood cholesterol, high
Deep Health®

Blood cleanser
Essiac Tonic
Liver Tonic™

Blood poisoning
Echinacea Triple Source™
Lymphatonic™
Phytocillin®

Blood pressure, high
HB Pressure™ Tonic

Blood sugar, low
Adrenotonic™

Blood triglycerides, high
Adrenotonic™
Deep Health®

Boils
Lymphatonic™
Phytocillin® (externally & internally)

Bone health
Menopautonic™

Bowel health
ParaFree™

Bronchiole health
Lung Tonic™
Respiratonic®

Bronchitis, acute
Peak Defense™
Phytocillin®
Respiratonic®

Bronchitis, chronic
Lung Tonic™

Bronchospasms
Lung Tonic™
Respiratonic®

Burns, skin
Lymphatonic™
Phytocillin®

Bursitis
Herbaprofen®

Cancer, support during treatment
Deep Health®
Essiac Tonic

Candidiasis (candida)
Phytocillin®
Yeast *ReLeaf*®

Canker sores
Mouth Tonic™

Cat scratch fever
Lymphatonic™

Catarrh (excess mucus)
Peak Defense™

Chemical exposure
Liver Tonic™

Chest cold
Immune Alert™
Peak Defense™
Phytocillin®
Respiratonic®

Cholesterol, elevated
Deep Health®

Chronic fatigue immuno-dysfunction syndrome (CFIDS)
Adrenotonic™
Essiac Tonic

Chronic obstructive pulmonary disease (COPD)
ChlorOxygen®
Lung Tonic™

Cirrhosis
Liver Tonic™

Cleansing
Essiac Tonic
Liver Tonic™
Lymphatonic™

Colds, first day
Immune Alert™

Colds, prevention of
Deep Health®
Immune Alert™
ImmunoBoost™

Colds, unshakable
Lymphatonic™

Colic
Stomach Tonic™

Colitis
Stomach Tonic™

Common cold
Immune Alert™
Echinacea Triple Source™
Peak Defense™
Phytocillin®
Respiratonic®

Common cold, prevention of
Deep Health®
ImmunoBoost™

Concentration
Remember Now™

Congestion
Allergy *ReLeaf*® System
Allertonic®
Congest Free™
Respiratonic®

Conjunctivitis
Allergy *ReLeaf*® System
Allertonic®

Constipation
Liver Tonic™

Convalescence
Adrenotonic™
Deep Health®
Ultimate Ginseng™

Coughs
Osha Root Throat Syrup
Respiratonic®
Singer's Saving Grace®

Cramps, intestinal
Herbaprofen®
Stomach Tonic™

Health Condition Index 111

Cramps, menstrual
  Cramp *ReLeaf*®
  Herbaprofen®

Cuts, infected
  Phytocillin®

Cuts, slow healing
  Deep Health®
  Lymphatonic™

Cystitis
  CranBladder *ReLeaf*®
  Kidney Tonic™

Cysts, breast, ovarian or uterine
  Lymphatonic™

Cytomegalovirus infection
  Deep Health®

Debility
  Adrenotonic™
  Deep Health®

Decubitus (bedsores)
  Lymphatonic™
    (internally)
  Phytocillin®
    (externally)

Dentures, sores from
  Mouth Tonic™

Deodorizer, intestinal
  ChlorOxygen®

Depression
  Deprezac™

Depression, with anxiety
  Kava Cool Complex™

Dermatitis
  Lymphatonic™

Diarrhea
  ParaFree™
  Yeast *ReLeaf*®

Diuretic
  Kidney Tonic™

Drug therapy, support during
  Adrenotonic™
  Deep Health®

Duodenal ulcers
  Stomach Tonic™

Dysentery
  ParaFree™

Dyspepsia
  Stomach Tonic™

Ears
  Mullein Garlic
    Ear Drops

Earache, from congestion
  Congest Free™
  Peak Defense™

Ear infection
  Peak Defense™
  Mullein Garlic
    Ear Drops
  Phytocillin®

Ear infection, recurrent
  Lymphatonic™
  Osha
  Phytocillin®

Emphysema
  Lung Tonic™

Endurance, lack of
  Adrenotonic™
  Deep Health®

Energy
  Adrenotonic™
  Deep Health®
  Ultimate Ginseng™
  Vibrant Energy™

Entamoeba
  ParaFree™

Enteritis
  Stomach Tonic™

Epstein-Barr virus
  Astragalus
  Deep Health®
  ImmunoBoost™

Exhaustion
Adrenotonic™
Deep Health®
Stress *ReLeaf*®
Ultimate Ginseng™

Expectorant
Osha Root Throat Syrup
Respiratonic®

Eye health
Allergy *ReLeaf*® System
Allertonic®

Eyes, mild infection
Phytocillin® (externally, diluted & internally)

Fasting
Lymphatonic™

Fatigue
Adrenotonic™
Deep Health®
Ultimate Ginseng™
Vibrant Energy™

Fatty liver
Liver Tonic™

Fermentation, intestinal
Stomach Tonic™

Fertility, low male
Prostatonic™

Fever
Herbaprofen®
Peak Defense™

Fibroid cysts, breast, uterine, ovarian
Lymphatonic™

Fibromyalgia
Herbaprofen®

Fibrositis
Arthrotonic™
Herbaprofen®

Flatulence
Stomach Tonic™

Flu
Immune Alert™
Loviral™
Peak Defense™

Fungal infection
Phytocillin®
Yeast *ReLeaf*®

Gallbladder
Liver Tonic™

Gallstones, mild
Herbaprofen®
Liver Tonic™

Gas
Stomach Tonic™

Gastric ulcers
Stomach Tonic™

Gastritis/gastroenteritis
Stomach Tonic™

Giardial infection
ParaFree™

Gingivitis
Mouth Tonic™

Gout
Lymphatonic™

Gum disease
Mouth Tonic™

Gum inflammation
Mouth Tonic™

Hay fever
Adrenotonic™
Allergy *ReLeaf*® System
Allertonic®

Hay fever, prevention of
Adrenotonic™
Allergy *ReLeaf*® System
Allertonic®
Deep Health®

Head cold
Congest Free™
Peak Defense™

Headache, acute
Herbaprofen®
Migra-Free®

Health Condition Index 113

Headache, chronic
Liver Tonic™
Migra-Free®

Heartburn
Stomach Tonic™

Heart palpitations (menopausal)
Adrenotonic™
Menopautonic™

Heart tonic
Deep Health®

Hepatitis
Deep Health®
Liver Tonic™

Herpes
Echinacea Triple Source™
Lymphatonic™
Mouth Tonic™

Hiccups
Stomach Tonic™

High altitude sickness
ChlorOxygen®

High blood pressure
HB Pressure™ Tonic

Hives
Allergy *ReLeaf*® System
Allertonic®
Ivy Itch ReLeaf® (externally)

Hoarseness
Singer's Saving Grace®

Hot flashes
Adrenotonic™
Menopautonic™

Hypersecretion of mucus
Allergy *ReLeaf*® System
Allertonic®
Peak Defense™

Hypertension
HB Pressure™ Tonic

Hypochondria
Adrenotonic™
Deep Health®
Nervine Tonic™

Hypoglycemia
Adrenotonic™

Illness, recuperating from
Deep Health®
Lymphatonic™

Immune system health
Deep Health®
Immune Alert™
ImmunoBoost™
Lymphatonic™

Immune system stimulation
Echinacea Triple Source™
ImmunoBoost™
Lymphatonic™

Immune system tonic
Deep Health®
ImmunoBoost™

Immune system, lingering or recurring illness
Lymphatonic™
Phytocillin®

Impetigo
Immune Alert™
Lymphatonic™
Phytocillin® (externally & internally)

Impotence
Prostatonic™

Indigestion
Stomach Tonic™

Infants, colic
Stomach Tonic™

Infection
Immune Alert™
Phytocillin®

114 CHAPTER 9

Infection, recurring
Lymphatonic™
Phytocillin®

Inflammation, gastrointestinal
Stomach Tonic™

Inflammation, joints
Herbaprofen®

Insect bites
Bug Itch *ReLeaf*® (externally)
Immune Alert™ (externally & internally)
Echinacea Triple Source™ (externally & internally)
Lymphatonic™ (internally)

Insomnia
Deep Sleep®
Kava Cool Complex™
Nervine Tonic™
Stress *ReLeaf*®

Intercourse, painful
Menopautonic™

Intercourse, urinary infection after
CranBladder *ReLeaf*®
Kidney Tonic™

Interferon, production of
Astragalus
Deep Health®
Echinacea Triple Source™
ImmunoBoost™

Intestinal distress
ParaFree™
Stomach Tonic™

Irritable bowel syndrome
Deep Health®
Stomach Tonic™

Jaundice
Liver Tonic™

Jaw, tense
Kava Cool Complex™
Nervine Tonic™
Stress *ReLeaf*®

Joint health
Herbaprofen®

Kidney infection
Kidney Tonic™

Laryngitis
Osha Root Throat Syrup
Singer's Saving Grace®

Leaky bowel syndrome
ParaFree™
Yeast *ReLeaf*®

Leukocyte, stimulation
Deep Health®
ImmunoBoost™

Leukorrhea
Immune Alert™
Yeast *ReLeaf*®

Lichen, infection
Phytocillin®
Yeast *ReLeaf*®

Ligament support
Echinacea Triple Source™

Liver support
Liver Tonic™

Lungs, congested
Osha Root Throat Syrup
Respiratonic®

Lungs, weak
Deep Health®
Lung Tonic™

Lupus, support in
Deep Health®
Lymphatonic™

Lymph nodes, swollen
Echinacea Triple Source™
Lymphatonic™

Health Condition Index

Lymphatic drainage
Lymphatonic™

Lymphedema
Lymphatonic™

Menopause
Adrenotonic™
Menopautonic™

Menstrual cramps
Cramp *ReLeaf*®

Menstrual migraine headaches
Migra-Free®

Metabolism, to balance
Adrenotonic™
Deep Health®

Metabolism, to stimulate
Vibrant Energy™

Metal, (heavy), exposure
Liver Tonic™

Middle ear infection
ImmunoBoost™
Mullein Garlic Ear Drops
Peak Defense™
Phytocillin®

Middle ear infection (recurring)
ImmunoBoost™
Lymphatonic™

Migraine headache
Migra-Free®

Miscarriage, prevention of
Cramp *ReLeaf*®

Mononucleosis
Liver Tonic™

Mood elevator
Deprezac™
Kava Cool Complex™
Stress *ReLeaf*®

Morning sickness
Cramp *ReLeaf*®

Mouth & gum health
Mouth Tonic™

Mucous membrane health
Allergy *ReLeaf*® System
Allertonic®

Mucus, excess
Peak Defense™
Respiratonic®

Mucus, lack of
Congest Free™

Muscle pain
Herbaprofen®

Muscle tension support
Kava Cool Complex™
Nervine Tonic™
Stress *ReLeaf*®

Myositis
Herbaprofen®

Nausea
Stomach Tonic™

Nephritis
Kidney Tonic™

Nervousness
Kava Cool Complex™
Nervine Tonic™
Stress *ReLeaf*®

Nervous system, exhaustion
Adrenotonic™
Deep Health®
Nervine Tonic™
Stress *ReLeaf*®

Nervous system, hyperactivity
Nervine Tonic™
Stress *ReLeaf*®

Neuralgia
Herbaprofen®
Nervine Tonic™
Stress *ReLeaf*®

Neuritis
Herbaprofen®
Nervine Tonic™
Stress *ReLeaf*®

Nicotine withdrawal
Nervine Tonic™
Smoke Free®
Stress *ReLeaf*®

Opiate withdrawal
Adrenotonic™
Stress *ReLeaf*®

Oral health
Mouth Tonic™

Otitis media, acute
Lymphatonic™
Mullein Garlic Ear Drops
Peak Defense™
Phytocillin®

Otitis media, prevention of
ImmunoBoost™
Lymphatonic™

Ovarian cyst
Lymphatonic™

Overexertion, muscle pain from
Herbaprofen®
Stress *ReLeaf*®

Pain
Herbaprofen®
Nervine Tonic™
Stress *ReLeaf*®

Pancreas health
Deep Health®

Panic attack
Deprezac™
Kava Cool Complex™
Stress *ReLeaf*®

Parasite cleanse
ParaFree™
Yeast *ReLeaf*®

Parasitic infection
ParaFree™

Peptic ulcer
Stomach Tonic™

Periodontal disease
Mouth Tonic™

Phantom pains
Nervine Tonic™

Pharyngitis
Singer's Saving Grace®

Pimples
Lymphatonic™

Pinworms
ParaFree™

Pleurisy
Loviral™
Phytocillin®
Respiratonic®

Pneumonia
Loviral™
Phytocillin®
Respiratonic®

Poison ivy/oak
Echinacea Triple Source™
Ivy Itch ReLeaf® (externally)
Lymphatonic™

Postpartum hemorrhage
Cramp *ReLeaf*®

PMS, water retention from
Kidney Tonic™

Prostatitis
Prostatonic™

Protozoal infection
ParaFree™

Psoriasis
Liver Tonic™

Pyorrhea
Mouth Tonic™

Health Condition Index

Red blood cells, low
ChlorOxygen®

Rejuvenation
Adrenotonic™
Deep Health®
Stress *ReLeaf*®
Ultimate Ginseng™

Relaxation
Kava Cool Complex™
Nervine Tonic™
Stress *ReLeaf*®

Respiratory system support
ChlorOxygen®
Deep Health®
Lung Tonic™
Respiratonic®

Restlessness
Kava Cool Complex™
Nervine Tonic™
Stress *ReLeaf*®

Rheumatic arthritis
Herbaprofen®

Rhinitis
Allergy *ReLeaf*® System
Allertonic®
Congest Free™

Ringworm
Yeast *ReLeaf*®

Sciatica
Herbaprofen®
Nervine Tonic™

Seasonal affective disorder (SAD)
Deprezac™

Sedative
Deep Sleep®
Kava Cool Complex™
Nervine Tonic™

Sexual tonic for men
Deep Health®

Sexual tonic for women
Deep Health®

Shingles
Herbaprofen®
Nervine Tonic™
Stress *ReLeaf*®

Sinusitis
Allergy *ReLeaf*® System
Allertonic®
Congest Free™
Loviral™

Skin health
Phytocillin®

Skin, sores
Lymphatonic™

Sleeping, excessive
Deep Health®
Deprezac™

Sleeping, problems
Deep Sleep®
Kava Cool Complex™
Stress *ReLeaf*®

Smoking, withdrawal from
Adrenotonic™
Smoke Free®
Stress *ReLeaf*®

Solvent exposure
Liver Tonic™

Sore throat
Osha Root Throat Syrup
Respiratonic®
Singer's Saving Grace®

Spasms, muscles
Herbaprofen®
Nervine Tonic™
Stress *ReLeaf*®

Spider bites
Bug Itch *ReLeaf*® (externally)
Echinacea Triple Source™ (externally & internally)

Splenitis
Lymphatonic™

Sprain
Herbaprofen®

Staph infection
Peak Defense™
Phytocillin®

Steroids, withdrawal from
Adrenotonic™

Stimulant
Vibrant Energy™

Stings, insects
Bug Itch *ReLeaf*®
(externally)
Echinacea Triple
Source™ (externally
& internally)
Ivy Itch ReLeaf®
(externally)

Stomach inflammation
Stomach Tonic™

Stomach support
Stomach Tonic™

Stones, gallbladder
Liver Tonic™

Strain
Herbaprofen®

Strep infection
Phytocillin®

Stress support
Adrenotonic™
Deep Health®
Kava Cool Complex™
Nervine Tonic™
Stress *ReLeaf*®

Stye
Immune Alert™
Lymphatonic™

Surgery, recuperating from
Adrenotonic™
Deep Health®

Swelling
Echinacea Triple
Source™
Lymphatonic™

Synovial inflammation
Herbaprofen®

Tendonitis
Echinacea Triple
Source™
Herbaprofen®

Tennis elbow
Echinacea Triple
Source™
Herbaprofen®

Tension
Kava Cool Complex™
Nervine Tonic™
Stress *ReLeaf*®

Testosterone, excessively low
Prostatonic™

Throat, sore
Osha Root Throat Syrup
Respiratonic®
Singer's Saving Grace®

Throat, strep
Loviral™
Peak Defense™
Phytocillin®

Thrush
Mouth Tonic™
Phytocillin®
Yeast *ReLeaf*®

Tiredness
Adrenotonic™
Deep Health®
Vibrant Energy™

Tonic, general
Deep Health®
Ultimate Ginseng™

Tonsillitis
Lymphatonic™
Phytocillin®

Health Condition Index

Toothache
Herbaprofen®

Tranquilizer
Kava Cool Complex™
Nervine Tonic™

Trichomoniasis
Lymphatonic™
Yeast *ReLeaf*®

Triglycerides, high
Ultimate Ginseng™

Tumors, benign
Deep Health®
Essiac Tonic

Twitching, muscle
Nervine Tonic™
Stress *ReLeaf*®

Ulceration
Phytocillin®

Urethritis
CranBladder *ReLeaf*®
Kidney Tonic™

Uric acid, to decrease
Lymphatonic™

Urinary tract infection (UTI)
CranBladder *ReLeaf*®
Kidney Tonic™

Urticaria
Allergy *ReLeaf*® System
Allertonic®
Lymphatonic™

Uterine cysts (fibroids)
Lymphatonic™

Uterine support
Cramp *ReLeaf*®

Vagina, dry
Adrenotonic™
Menopautonic™

Viral infection
Immune Alert™
Loviral™
Phytocillin®

Vitality, low
Adrenotonic™
Deep Health®
Ultimate Ginseng™

Vomiting
Stomach Tonic™

Warts
Phytocillin®
Yeast *ReLeaf*®

Water retention
Kidney Tonic™

Weakness
Adrenotonic™
Deep Health®

White blood cells, low
Echinacea Triple Source™
ImmunoBoost™
Lymphatonic™

Women's health
CranBladder *ReLeaf*®
Cramp *ReLeaf*®
Menopautonic™
Yeast *ReLeaf*®

Wound
Phytocillin®

Yeast infection
Phytocillin®
Yeast *ReLeaf*®

Chapter 10

Common Name–Latin Name Index

Use this index to find or learn the Latin name of a particular herb. The first word of the latin name denotes the genus of the herb while the second word denotes the species. Sometimes the words "et al." follow the Latin name. These two words simply mean "and others" and indicate that other species of same genus can be used interchangeably with the species listed. For example, *Euphrasia stricta* can be substituted for *Euphrasia roskoviana.* Both species are known to be interchangeable and are as effective as one another.

Common Name	Latin Name
Andrographis	*Andrographis paniculata*
Angelica	*Angelica archangelica*
Ashwagandha	*Withania somnifera*
Astragalus	*Astragalus membranaceus*
Balsam poplar	*Populus balsamifera*
Bayberry	*Morella pensylvanica*
Bethroot	*Trillium erectum*
Betony	*Pedicularis canadensis* et al.
Black cherry	*Prunus serotina*
Black cohosh	*Actaea racemosa*
Black currant	*Ribes nigrum*
Black haw	*Viburnum prunifolium*
Black walnut	*Juglans nigra*
Bloodroot	*Sanguinaria canadensis*
Blue flag	*Iris versicolor* et al.
Boldo	*Peumus boldus*
Buchu	*Agathosma betulina* et al.
Burdock	*Arctium lappa*
Calendula	*Calendula officinalis*
California poppy	*Eschscholzia californica*
California spikenard	*Aralia californica*
Cardamom	*Elettaria cardamomum*
Cassia	*Cinnamomum aromaticum*
Catnip	*Nepeta cataria*
Cayenne	*Capsicum annuum*
Celandine	*Chelidonium majus*
Chamomile	*Matricaria recutita*
Chaste tree	See Vitex

Health Condition Index 121

Chinese lovage	*Ligusticum jeholense* et al.
Chinese mint	*Mentha canadensis*
Chinese (Turkey) rhubarb	*Rheum officinale*
Cinnamon	*Cinnamomum verum*
Cleavers	*Galium aparine*
Clove	*Syzygium aromaticum*
Cordyceps	*Cordyceps sinensis* et al.
Couch grass	*Elymus repens*
Cramp bark	*Viburnum opulus*
Cranberry	*Vaccinium macrocarpon*
Cubeb	*Piper cubeba*
Culver's root	*Veronicastrum virginicum*
Damiana	*Turnera diffusa*
Dandelion	*Taraxacum officinale*
Devil's claw	*Harpagophytum procumbens*
Dong quai	*Angelica sinensis*
Echinacea angustifolia	*Echinacea angustifolia*
Echinacea pallida	*Echinacea pallida*
Echinacea purpurea	*Echinacea purpurea*
Elder	*Sambucus nigra* et al.
Elecampane	*Inula helenium*
Eleuthero, Siberian	*Eleutherococcus senticosus*
European mistletoe	*Viscum album*
Eyebright	*Euphrasia rostkoviana* et al.
Fennel	*Foeniculum vulgare*
Feverfew	*Tanacetum parthenium*
Fo-ti	*Polygonum multiflorum*
Fringe tree	*Chionanthus virginicus*
Garlic	*Allium sativum*
Gentian	*Gentiana lutea*
Ginger	*Zingiber officinale*
Ginkgo	*Ginkgo biloba*
Ginseng, American, cultivated	*Panax quinquefolius*
Ginseng, American, wild	*Panax quinquefolius*
Ginseng, American, woodsgrown	*Panax quinquefolius*
Ginseng, Asian, red kirin	*Panax ginseng*
Ginseng, Asian, white	*Panax ginseng*
Goldenseal	*Hydrastis canadensis*
Gotu kola	*Centella asiatica*

Graviola	*Annona muricata*
Grindelia	*Grindelia camporum* et al.
Hawthorn	*Crataegus monogyna* et al.
Holy basil (Krishna and Rama tulsi)	*Ocimum tenuiflorum*
Honeysuckle	*Lonicera confusa* et al.
Hops	*Humulus lupulus*
Horehound	*Marrubium vulgare*
Horsetail	*Equisetum arvense*
Jack-in-the-pulpit	*Arisaema triphyllum*
Jamaica dogwood	*Piscidia piscipula*
Jewel weed	*Impatiens capensis* et al.
Juniper	*Juniperus communis*
Kava	*Piper methysticum*
Lavender	*Lavandula angustifolia* et al.
Lemon balm	*Melissa officinalis*
Lesser periwinkle	*Vinca minor*
Licorice	*Glycyrrhiza glabra*
Linden	*Tilia cordata* et al.
Lobelia	*Lobelia inflata*
Lomatium	*Lomatium dissectum*
Magnolia	*Magnolia acuminata* et al.
Maitake	*Grifola frondosa*
Male fern	*Dryopteris filix-mas*
Meadowsweet	*Filipendula ulmaria*
Milk thistle	*Silybum marianum*
Motherwort	*Leonurus cardiaca*
Mullein	*Verbascum thapsus*
Myrrh	*Commiphora myrrha* et al.
Oat	*Avena sativa*
Ocotillo	*Fouquieria splendens*
Olive	*Olea europaea*
Orange	*Citrus sinensis*
Oregon grape	*Mahonia aquifolium* et al.
Osha	*Ligusticum porteri*
Parsley	*Petroselinum crispum*
Passionflower	*Passiflora incarnata*
Pau d'arco	*Tabebuia impetiginosa*
Pelargonium	*Pelargonium sidoides* (*umckaloabo*) et al.
Peppermint	*Mentha* x *piperita*
Pipsissewa	*Chimaphila umbellata*
Plantain	*Plantago major*
Pleurisy root	*Asclepias tuberosa*
Prickly ash	*Zanthoxylum americanum*
Quassia	*Quassia amara*
Red root	*Ceanothus americanus* et al.

Health Condition Index 123

Reishi	*Ganoderma lucidum*
Rosemary	*Rosmarinus officinalis*
Sarsaparilla	*Smilax febrifuga* et al.
Saw palmetto	*Serenoa repens*
Schisandra	*Schisandra chinensis* et al.
Sheep sorrel	*Rumex acetosella*
Shiitake	*Lentinula edodes*
Skullcap	*Scutellaria lateriflora*
Slippery elm	*Ulmus rubra*
Spikenard	*Aralia racemosa*
Spilanthes	*Spilanthes oleracea* et al.
St. John's wort	*Hypericum perforatum*
Star anise	*Illicium verum*
Stevia	*Stevia rebaudiana*
Stillingia	*Stillingia sylvatica*
Stinging nettle	*Urtica dioica* ssp. *dioica*
Stoneroot	*Collinsonia canadensis*
Thuja	*Thuja occidentalis*
Toadflax	*Linaria vulgaris* et al.
Turmeric	*Curcuma longa*
Usnea	*Usnea barbata*
Uva-ursi	*Arctostaphylos uva-ursi*
Valerian	*Valeriana officinalis*
Vitex	*Vitex agnus-castus*
White pine	*Pinus strobus*
White willow	*Salix alba*
Wild indigo	*Baptisia tinctoria*
Wild yam	*Dioscorea villosa*
Wormwood	*Artemisia absinthium*
Xanthium	*Xanthium sibiricum*
Yarrow	*Achillea millefolium*
Yellow dock	*Rumex crispus*
Yerba mansa	*Anemopsis californica*
Yerba santa	*Eriodictyon californicum* et al.

The two ingredients, Chlorophyll and Propolis, do not have Latin binomial names.

Chapter 11

Latin Name–Common Name Index

Use this index to find the common name of an herb. There have been numerous times when common names have been used to identify more than one herb. Botanists use Latin names because each Latin name identifies one specific herb only. However, there are some herbs from the same species that can be used interchangeably. For example: *Agathosma betulina* (short buchu), *Agathosma crenulata* (ovate buchu) and *Agathosma serratifolia* (long buchu) are so similar that all three species are used interchangeably. That's why "et al." is used after *Agathosma betulina*; it means "and others."

Latin Name	**Common**
Achillea millefolium	Yarrow
Actaea racemosa	Black cohosh
Agathosma betulina et al.	Buchu
Allium sativum	Garlic
Andrographis paniculata	Andrographis
Anemopsis californica	Yerba mansa
Angelica archangelica	Angelica
Angelica sinensis	Dong quai
Aralia californica	California spikenard
Aralia racemosa	Spikenard
Arctium lappa	Burdock
Arctostaphylos uva-ursi	Uva-ursi
Arisaema triphyllum	Jack-in-the-pulpit
Artemisia absinthium	Wormwood
Asclepias tuberosa	Pleurisy root
Astragalus membranaceus	Astragalus
Avena sativa	Oat
Baptisia tinctoria	Wild indigo
Calendula officinalis	Calendula
Capsicum annuum	Cayenne
Ceanothus americanus et al.	Red root
Centella asiatica	Gotu kola
Chelidonium majus	Celandine
Chimaphila umbellata	Pipsissewa
Chionanthus virginicus	Fringe tree
Cinnamomum aromaticum	Cassia

Health Condition Index 125

Cinnamomum verum	Cinnamon
Citrus sinensis	Orange
Collinsonia canadensis	Stoneroot
Commiphora myrrha et al.	Myrrh
Cordyceps sinensis et al.	Cordyceps
Crataegus monogyna et al.	Hawthorn
Curcuma longa	Turmeric
Dioscorea villosa	Wild yam
Dryopteris filix-mas	Male fern
Echinacea angustifolia	*Echinacea angustifolia*
Echinacea pallida	*Echinacea pallida*
Echinacea purpurea	*Echinacea purpurea*
Elettaria cardamomum	Cardamom
Eleutherococcus senticosus	Eleuthero, Siberian
Elymus repens	Couch grass
Equisetum arvense	Horsetail
Eriodictyon californicum et al.	Yerba santa
Eschscholzia californica	California poppy
Euphrasia rostkoviana et al.	Eyebright
Filipendula ulmaria	Meadowsweet
Foeniculum vulgare	Fennel
Fouquieria splendens	Ocotillo
Galium aparine	Cleavers
Ganoderma lucidum	Reishi
Gentiana lutea	Gentian
Ginkgo biloba	Ginkgo
Glycyrrhiza glabra	Licorice
Grifola frondosa	Maitake
Grindelia camporum et al.	Grindelia
Harpagophytum procumbens	Devil's claw
Humulus lupulus	Hops
Hydrastis canadensis	Goldenseal
Hypericum perforatum	St. John's wort
Illicium verum	Star anise
Impatiens capensis et al.	Jewel weed
Inula helenium	Elecampane
Iris versicolor et al.	Blue flag
Juglans nigra	Black walnut
Juniperus communis	Juniper
Lavandula angustifolia et al.	Lavender
Lentinula edodes	Shiitake
Leonurus cardiaca	Motherwort
Ligusticum jeholense et al.	Chinese lovage
Ligusticum porteri	Osha
Linaria vulgaris et al.	Toadflax

Lobelia inflata	Lobelia
Lomatium dissectum	Lomatium
Lonicera confusa et al.	Honeysuckle
Magnolia acuminata et al.	Magnolia
Mahonia aquifolium et al.	Oregon grape
Marrubium vulgare	Horehound
Matricaria recutita	Chamomile
Melissa officinalis	Lemon balm
Mentha canadensis	Chinese mint
Mentha x piperita	Peppermint
Morella pensylvanica	Bayberry
Nepeta cataria	Catnip
Ocimum tenuiflorum	Holy basil (Krishna and Rama tulsi)
Olea europaea	Olive
Panax ginseng	Ginseng, Asian, red kirin
Panax ginseng	Ginseng, Asian, white
Panax quinquefolius	Ginseng, American, cultivated
Panax quinquefolius	Ginseng, American, wild
Panax quinquefolius	Ginseng, American, woodsgrown
Passiflora incarnata	Passionflower
Pedicularis canadensis et al.	Betony
Pelargonium sidoides (*umckaloabo*) et al.	Pelargonium
Petroselinum crispum	Parsley
Peumus boldus	Boldo
Pinus strobus	White pine
Piper cubeba	Cubeb
Piper methysticum	Kava
Piscidia piscipula	Jamaica dogwood
Plantago major	Plantain
Polygonum multiflorum	Fo-ti
Populus balsamifera	Balsam poplar
Prunus serotina	Black cherry
Quassia amara	Quassia
Rheum officinale	Chinese (Turkey) rhubarb
Ribes nigrum	Black currant
Rosmarinus officinalis	Rosemary
Rumex acetosella	Sheep sorrel
Rumex crispus	Yellow dock
Salix alba	White willow
Sambucus nigra et al.	Elder

Sanguinaria canadensis	Bloodroot
Schisandra chinensis et al.	Schisandra
Scutellaria lateriflora	Skullcap
Serenoa repens	Saw palmetto
Silybum marianum	Milk thistle
Smilax febrifuga et al.	Sarsaparilla
Spilanthes oleracea et al.	Spilanthes
Stevia rebaudiana	Stevia
Stillingia sylvatica	Stillingia
Syzygium aromaticum	Clove
Tabebuia impetiginosa	Pau d'arco
Tanacetum parthenium	Feverfew
Taraxacum officinale	Dandelion
Thuja occidentalis	Thuja
Tilia cordata et al.	Linden
Trillium erectum	Bethroot
Turnera diffusa	Damiana
Ulmus rubra	Slippery elm
Urtica dioica ssp. *dioica*	Stinging nettle
Usnea barbata	Usnea
Vaccinium macrocarpon	Cranberry
Valeriana officinalis	Valerian
Verbascum thapsus	Mullein
Veronicastrum virginicum	Culver's root
Viburnum opulus	Cramp bark
Viburnum prunifolium	Black haw
Vinca minor	Lesser periwinkle
Viscum album	European mistletoe
Vitex agnus-castus	Vitex
Withania somnifera	Ashwagandha
Xanthium sibiricum	Xanthium
Zanthoxylum americanum	Prickly ash
Zingiber officinale	Ginger

The two ingredients, Chlorophyll and Propolis, do not have Latin binomial names.

et al. means "and others"

Suggested Reading

The following authors present useful and practical information for the person interested in herbs, herbal medicine, and health.

Daniel Gagnon and Amadea Morningstar

Breathe Free

This book was written because I wanted to share practical information on how to treat respiratory problems. My frustration with most existing herbal books is that they tell you which herbs to use, but not how much to take and why. Therefore, *Breathe Free* gives you specifics on which foods, supplements and herbs to take. It covers such problems as common colds and flu, hay fever, sore throats, earaches, asthma, pneumonia, bronchitis, emphysema, and more.

Christopher Hobbs

Echinacea, The Immune Herb
Foundations of Health
Handbook for Herbal Healing
Milk Thistle, The Liver Herb
Natural Liver Therapy
Medicinal Mushrooms
Usnea, The Herbal Antibiotic
Valerian, The Relaxing and Sleep Herb
Vitex, The Women's Herb

Christopher's books strike a good balance between imparting high-level scientific research and translating those research results into practical information for everyday use.

David Hoffmann

The New Holistic Herbal
An Elders' Herbal

If you buy just one other herbal book for your family (in addition to *The Practical Guide to Herbal Medicines*), I would strongly suggest that it be David's *The New Holistic Herbal*. Due to its comprehensive approach and well-organized chapters, I highly encourage my herbal medicine students to read this book cover to cover. It is chockfull with useful and practical information.

Michael Moore

> *Medicinal Plants of the Desert and Canyon West*
> *Medicinal Plants of the Mountain West*
> *Medicinal Plants of the Pacific West*

Michael's great sense of humor turns what could be the most potentially boring reading into an interesting and humorous experience. In his book *Medicinal Plants of the Pacific West*, for instance, his comparison of an herb called Western Skunk Cabbage to the carnivorous plant in the movie *Little Shop of Horrors* is funny yet informative. Michael's incredible unparalleled knowledge of physiology and profound understanding of the medicinal actions of herbs make his books required reading for anyone who is truly interested in herbal medicine.

Michael Tierra

> *The Way of Herbs*
> *Planetary Herbology*

The Way of Herbs is an excellent introduction to herbal medicine. *Planetary Herbology* is a fascinating, eclectic book incorporating Ayurvedic Medicine, Traditional Chinese Medicine and Western Herbology points of view.

Susun Weed

> *Breast Cancer? Breast Health! The Wise Woman Way*
> *Wise Woman Herbal: Healing Wise*
> *Wise Woman Herbal for the Childbearing Years*
> *Wise Woman Herbal for the Menopausal Years*

Susun's writings express strong opinions. Her books are directed toward empowering women to become involved in their own health care. I highly respect her work and recommend her books to those interested in expanding their women's health and herbal medicine horizons. Additionally, Susun's poetic side is evident in her work.

Suggested Reading

Additional reading for the serious student and the health professional.

American Herbal Products Association
Botanical Safety Handbook 2nd Edition (2012)

Bensky and Gamble
Chinese Herbal Medicine Materia Medica (1986)

Bone and Mills
Principles and Practice of Phytotherapy (2013)

Chen and Chen
Chinese Medical Herbology and Pharmacology (2001)

Finley Ellingwood
American Materia Medica, Therapeutics and Pharmacognosy (1986)
Although first published in 1898, the information in this book is still relevant.

Harvey Felter
The Eclectic Materia Medica, Pharmacology and Therapeutics (1983)
Although first published in 1922, the information in this book is still relevant.

Felter and Lloyd (1983)
King's American Dispensatory (1983)
Although first published in 1898, the information in this book is still relevant.

David Hoffmann
Medical Herbalism (2003)

Mills and Bone
The Essential Guide to Herbal Safety (2005)

Sebastian Pole
Ayurvedic Medicine: The Principles of Traditional Practice (2006)

Rudolf Weiss
Herbal Medicine, 1st Edition only* (1988)
*Do not buy the 2nd Edition since it has been revised after Dr. Weiss' death.

Notes: